a garden project workbook

the

scented garden

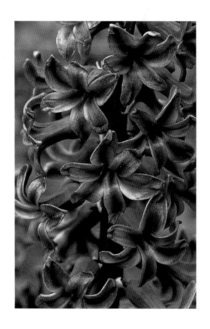

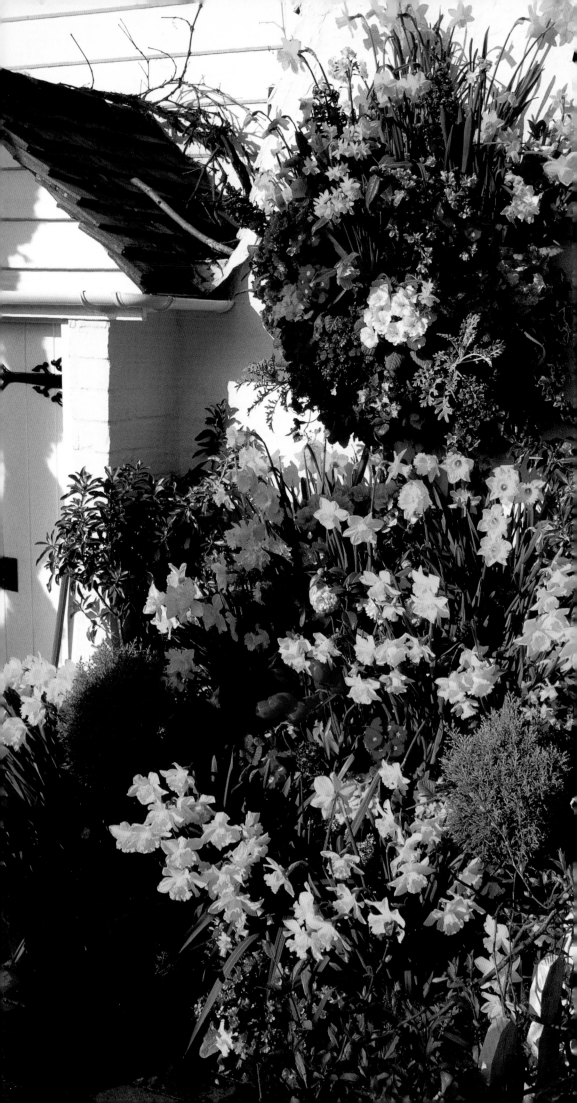

a garden project workbook

the
scented garden

Richard Bird

photography by **Jonathan Buckley**

STEWART, TABORI & CHANG
NEW YORK

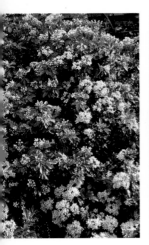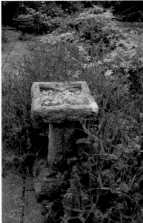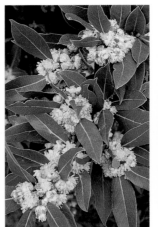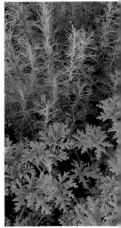

Text © 2000 Richard Bird
Photography © 2000 Jonathan Buckley

Design and photographs copyright
© 2000 Ryland Peters & Small

Published in 2000 by
Stewart, Tabori & Chang
A division of U.S. Media Holdings, Inc.
115 West 18th Street
New York, NY 10011

Distributed in Canada by
General Publishing Company Ltd
30 Lesmill Road
Don Mills, Ontario, Canada M3B 2T6

ISBN: 1-55670-961-7

A CIP catalogue record for this book is
available from the Library of Congress.

Produced in China by Sung Fung Offset
Binding Co., Ltd.

Composed in New Baskerville.
10 9 8 7 6 5 4 3 2 1
First Printing, 2000

Designed and edited by **cobalt id**

Illustration **Richard Bonson**

Project co-ordination **Paul Tilby**
Production **Meryl Silbert, Patricia Harrington**

Art Director **Gabriella Le Grazie**
Publishing Director **Anne Ryland**

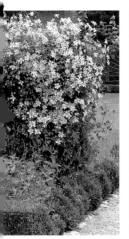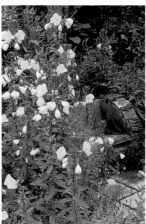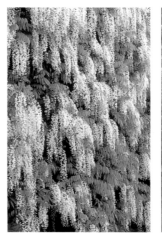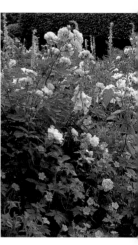

contents

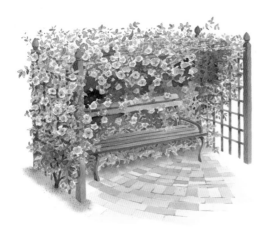

It is possible to create a garden without paying any attention to scent, and indeed many gardens are planned with exclusive regard for form and color. Yet to ignore scent is to remove the dimension that most enraptures any visitor to a garden; scent is the most evocative of our sensations, perhaps because it connects with parts of the brain that also handle emotion, and our childhood memories of gardens are typically anchored in scent rather than visual stimuli.

Gardens are perfumed both by flowers and foliage. Some scents are secret—the delicate perfumes of individual flowers must be sampled by a curious nose—while others are more public, filling the garden and creating a distinctive atmosphere across a wide area. Most fragrant foliage needs to be crushed or brushed against before it releases its scent and is well suited to paths and walks.

Scent is one of the greatest aids to relaxation in the garden. Try planting roses or other fragrant climbers over a framework under which you can sit and relax after work; night-scented climbers, such as honeysuckle and jasmine are ideally sited near open windows, or around areas in which you entertain during the long summer evenings.

Creating a fragrant garden is not difficult; this book introduces projects that will help you get the maximum benefit from the wide range of plants that form the scented garden. The plants given in the following plans and lists are suggestions only; please use your own favorites to create more personal gardens.

Richard Bird

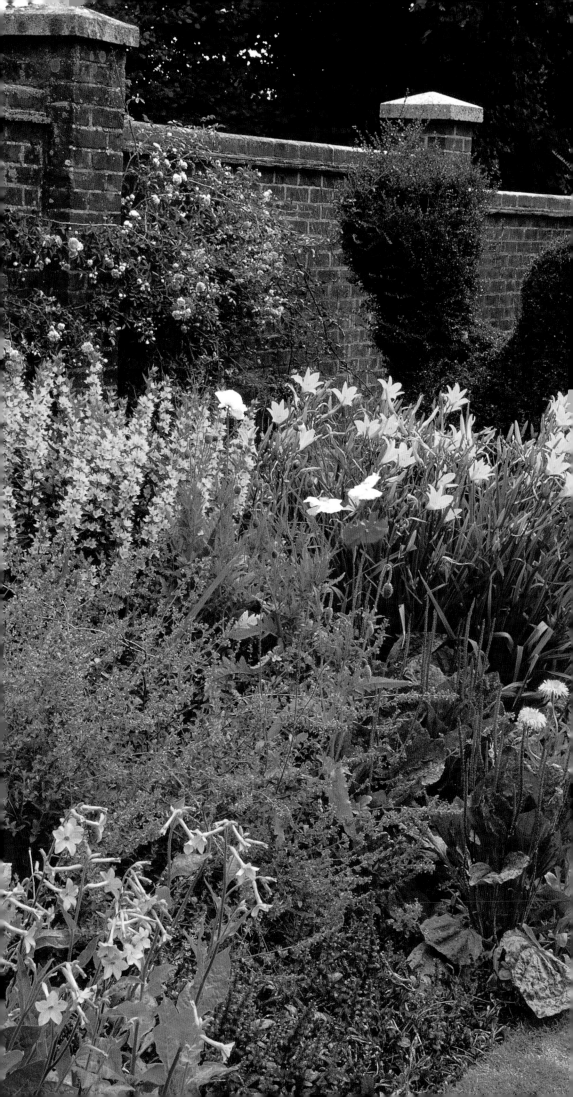

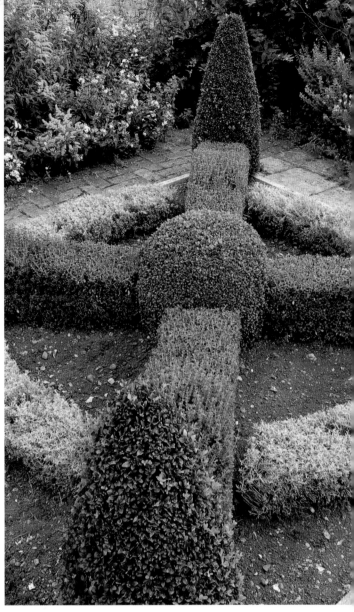

right In this parterre, or knot garden, the hedging is made up of scented santolina, teucrium, and box. The beds can be filled with scented plants, such as primulas or wallflowers in spring, and heliotrope in summer.

below A whole border can be filled with a single plant to great effect. Here catmint (*Nepeta*) produces a gray-blue haze of foliage and flowers. Similar borders can be created with with lavender or rosemary.

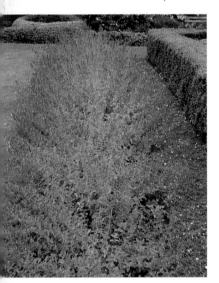

beds and borders are the mainstay of

gardens and it is here that most scented plants will be found growing with no special

treatment. However, these plants should be positioned with great care: they should

be well spaced to avoid clashes of scent—isolating each scent gives it the clarity it

deserves and makes a walk around the garden into an olfactory safari. Scented plants

should also be well spread out over the seasons so there is something to perfume the

garden during each month of the year.

right Rock gardens are not usually known for their scent. Raised areas between the rocks, however, are perfect for displaying smaller scented plants because it is easier to enjoy their fragrance at close quarters. The spread of plants should be controlled by regular pruning: mint (shown here), in particular, can become rampant.

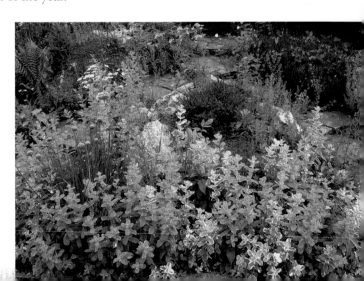

8

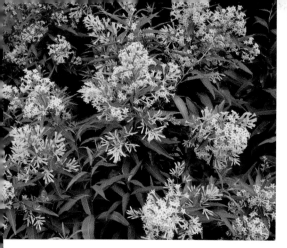

above The yellow flowers of *Cestrum parqui* are a curiosity among scented plants in that they have a savory smell during the day but give off a sweet scent in the evening. The decorative foliage and flowers are followed in autumn by purple berries.

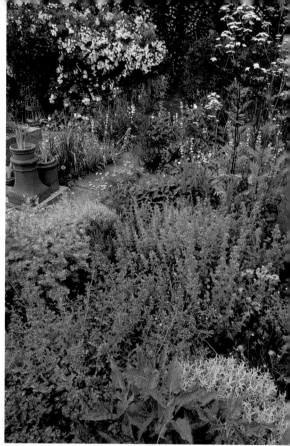

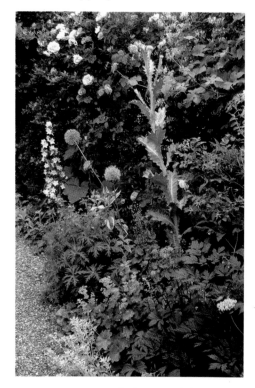

above Scent is not often associated with bright flowers – fragrant borders tend to be of more muted colors, as apparent here. If you want to brighten them up, add a few colorful but unscented plants.

left It is best to keep scents discrete by mixing plants that have scented flowers with those that have scented leaves and with unscented species. Here *Rosa* 'Albertine', *R.* 'Mrs. John Laing', and honeysuckle share space with lavender and unscented flowers.

below Lilies are ideal for the border—they mix well with both herbaceous and shrubby plants and have the most delicious scents, particularly on hot days. Remember to include a seat nearby.

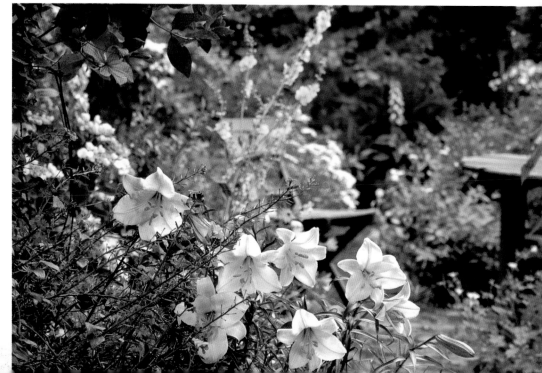

cutting border

Having cut flowers in the house is one of life's great pleasures, and growing your own adds greatly to that pleasure. Most gardens will provide enough cutting material for at least a posy, but for a regular supply it is a good idea to create your own cutting border where you can grow your favorite scented flowers. A separate border allows more attention to be given to growing quality blooms as well as preventing the main borders from being denuded when flowers are required.

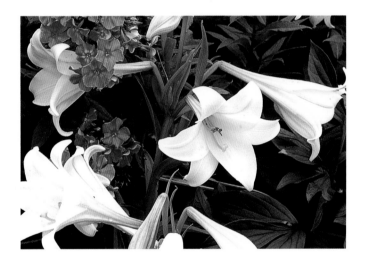

materials & equipment

spade
fork
rake
garden line or pegs and string
stakes
string
pruning shears
wooden mallet

plants in variety
well-rotted organic material

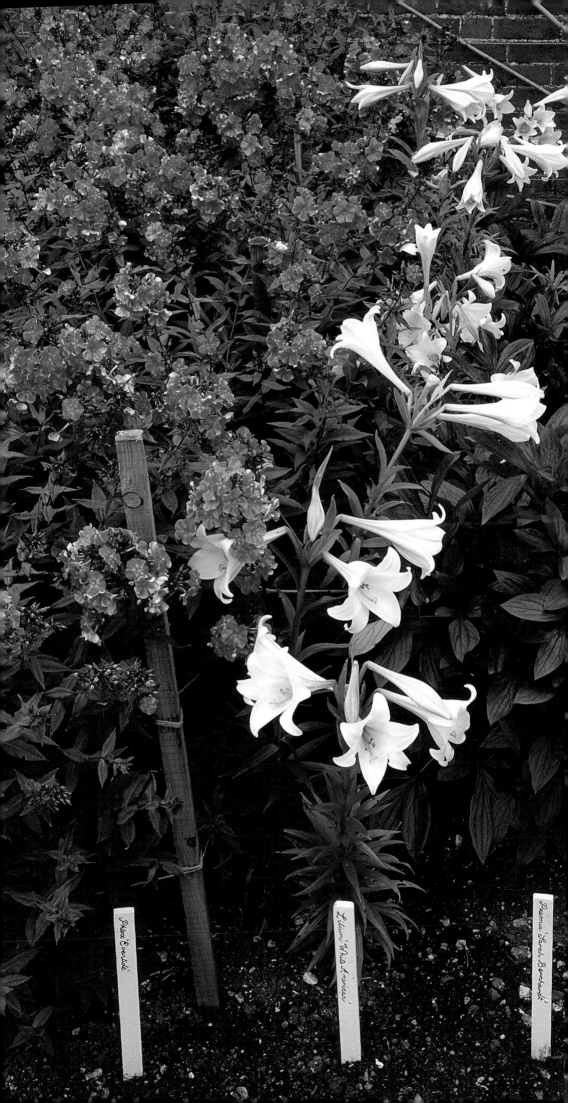

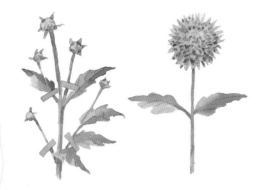

4 debudding

Many plants produce bigger and better blooms if they are debudded. This involves the removal of some of the flower buds so that the remaining ones fill out to their maximum size. This technique is used only with plants that can produce single heads, such as chrysanthemums or carnations; it would not be applied to the phlox and lilies in this planting.

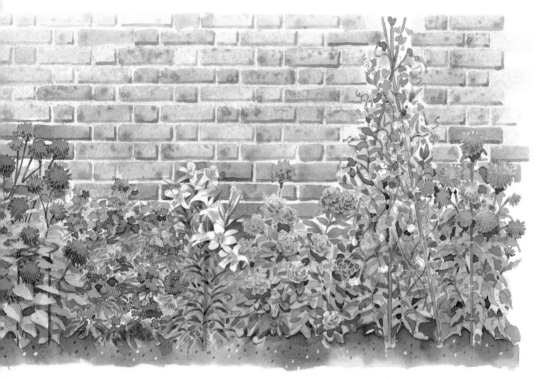

5 cutting the flowers

Cut the flowers when air temperature is cool, not when the plants are hot and flagging; early morning is best. Always cut with as long a stem as possible. If flowers are damaged, remove them from the plant.

6 preparing the flowers

Immediately after cutting, immerse the stem right up to the flower head in lukewarm water and stand in a cool place for several hours. This will condition the flower so that it later takes up water.

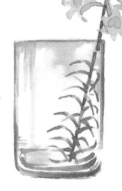

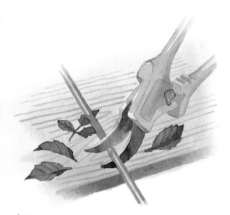

7 cutting for the vase

Trim the stems to the arranging length, cutting at an acute angle to present a greater surface to the water. Remove all of the foliage that will fall below the water line. Chemicals can be added to the water to prolong the cut flower's life.

plants with woody stems

Crush rather than cut the ends of woody plants, such as lilac (Syringa) and mock orange (Philadelphus).

1 preparing the ground

For the best blooms, the ground must be thoroughly prepared. Mark out the plot with string and pegs, and dig it deeply, incorporating as much well-rotted organic material as possible. This is best done in the autumn to be ready for spring planting. Any weeds that reappear in spring should be removed. Rake over the ground before planting to obtain a fine tilth.

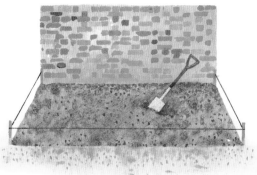

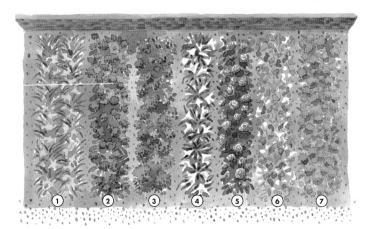

2 choosing the plants

Select plants that flower at different times of year to give a continuous supply of cutting material. Plant in rows at regular intervals, following the guidelines supplied with the seeds and bulbs. Leave at least 18 in (45 cm) between rows for maintenance and cutting.

plant list
1 *Narcissus* 'February Gold'
2 *Dahlia* (in variety)
3 *Phlox* 'Eventide'
4 *Lilium longiflorum* 'White American'
5 *Paeonia* 'Sarah Bernhardt'
6 *Lathyrus odoratus* (mixed colors)
7 *Chrysanthemum* (in variety)

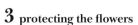

3 protecting the flowers

To reach perfection, cut flowers must be protected from the elements. Strong winds are capable of bruising flowers and breaking stems. If the plants are grown in rows, the simplest means of protection is to stake the whole row together using stakes or canes and string.

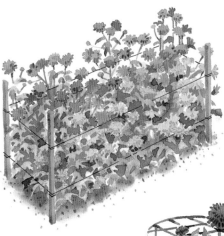

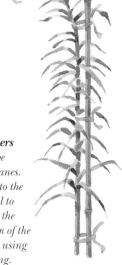

bushy plants

Clumps of plants can be protected from wind damage by using plant supports, such as hoops. These are most suitable for bushy plants with more than one stem.

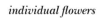

individual flowers

Tall plants can be supported with canes. Push the cane into the soil, being careful to avoid damaging the roots. Tie the stem of the plant to the cane using raffia or soft string.

11

rose garden

One of the basic ingredients of any scented garden is a rose bush. The height of sensuality is to have an entire garden devoted to roses and their delightful fragrances. A garden stretching for acres, with gardeners to look after it, is the ultimate, but for the average individual it is quite possible to create a small, intimate rose garden that will give just as much pleasure. This garden is filled with scented modern floribundas that flower over a long period.

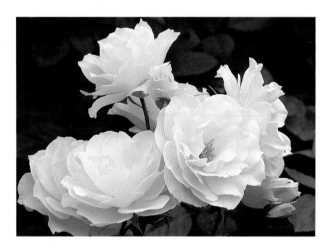

materials & equipment

4 paving slabs, 18 in x 2 ft (45 x 60 cm)
8 paving slabs 18 x 18 in (45 x 45 cm)
builder's sand
ornamental urn or sundial

pegs and string
two-foot square
tamper
spade
fork
trowel
rake
pruning shears

54 box plants (*Buxus sempervirens* 'Suffruticosa')
2 *Rosa* 'Saratoga'
2 *Rosa* 'Arthur Bell'
2 *Rosa* 'Elizabeth of Glamis'
well-rotted organic material

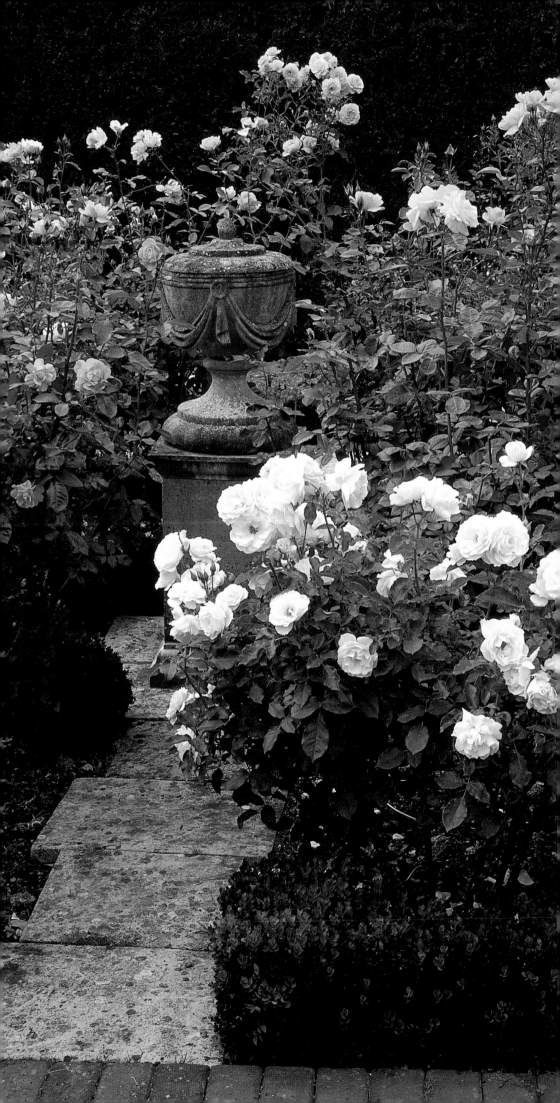

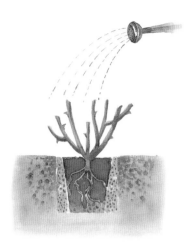

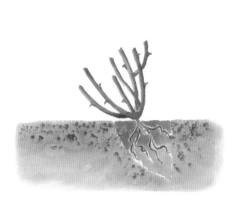

7 planting the roses

Dig a hole a little wider than the rootball of the plant. Bed in the rootball and fill in with good quality soil. Firm down and water. In windy areas, the plant will need a temporary stake. For bare-rooted plants, dig a wide hole and fan out the roots evenly around the plant before refilling with soil.

heeling in

Roses are one of the few plants that can still be purchased bare-rooted—without any soil around their roots. If they arrive when you cannot plant them in the desired places, store them by "heeling in." Dig a hole or trench and slip the plant in at an angle before refilling. Replant at a more convenient time. Stake before planting to avoid root damage.

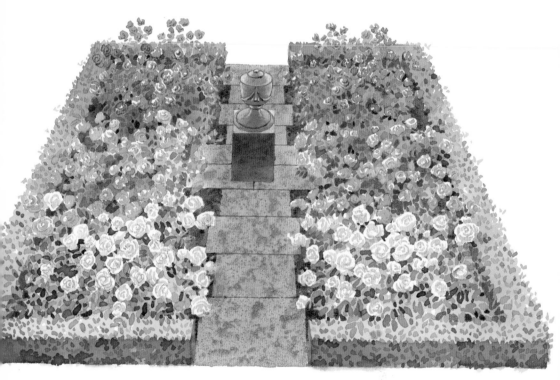

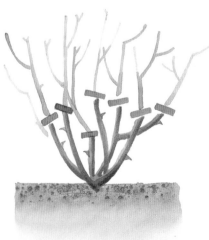

8 mature rose garden

The roses will take about two to three years to reach the size shown here. When the hedge gains the desired width and height, prune the leader and lateral shoots to keep it bushy.

9 pruning the roses

New bushes should be cut back to within about 3 in (8 cm) of the ground, pruning to an outward-facing bud. They should then be pruned every spring by cutting out any dead, dying, or spindly growth and reducing the rest to within 10 in (25 cm) of the ground, pruning to a strong outward-facing bud.

1 planning the layout

This plot is only 10 ft (3 m) square and so needs to be planned carefully. It's best to draw it out on paper. Your drawing should be roughly to scale so that you can work out how many roses you can fit into the space, and how they should best be arranged. This plan allows for a box hedge around the roses: this will help protect the young roses as well as providing an attractive geometrical border.

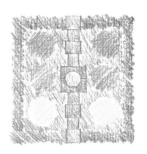

2 measuring out the plot

Transfer the outline of your plan to the ground. Place pegs in the ground to mark out the four corners; use string and a two-foot square to check that the corners are right angles. Find the center of the plot by pulling two strings across the diagonals—they cross at the geometric center. Mark this with a peg.

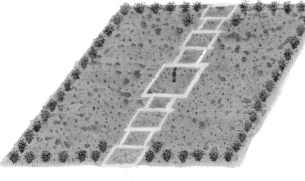

3 preparing the plot

In the autumn, dig well within the marked area, remove all weeds, and incorporate as much organic material as you can. If there are a lot of perennial weeds, kill them once and for all with an single application of chemical herbicide. Plant young box plants at 9 in (23 cm) intervals just within the dug area. Firm in, water, and keep watered in dry weather. Mark out the rough position of the path using pegs and string or sand poured from a bottle.

4 building the path

The path through the rose garden is made up of two sizes of paving slabs laid on compacted sand. Before laying the path, make certain that the soil beneath the slabs is well tamped down so that the slabs will not sink.

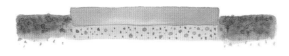

5 laying the slabs

Rake across the compacted soil surface to level it and then pour on a 2 in (5 cm) layer of soft builder's sand. Place the paving slabs on top and tamp them down so that they are level. On light, sandy soils the slabs can be bedded straight down onto the soil without an intermediate layer of sand.

6 arranging the path

The path is made up of alternating large and small slabs. The central area, where the urn is placed, is made up of four smaller slabs put together to make a 2 x 3 ft (60 x 90) rectangle.

aromatic mixed border

Planting a border with annuals alone is very restrictive. Mixing in scented perennials, annuals, shrubs, and even small trees adds interest and helps create a changing scene in which certain elements remain throughout the year, while others change week by week. The planting mixture should include a sprinkling of unscented species, otherwise the perfume of the border can become jumbled and overpowering; confining yourself to scented plants is also likely to restrict the visual impact of the border.

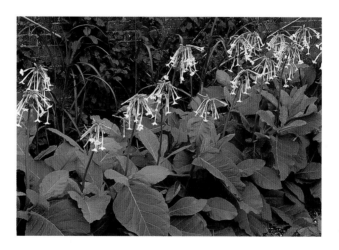

materials & equipment

graph paper
pencil and ruler
pegs and string
cold frame
light-colored sand
empty bottle

spade
fork
rake
trowel
pruning shears

plants in variety
well-rotted organic material

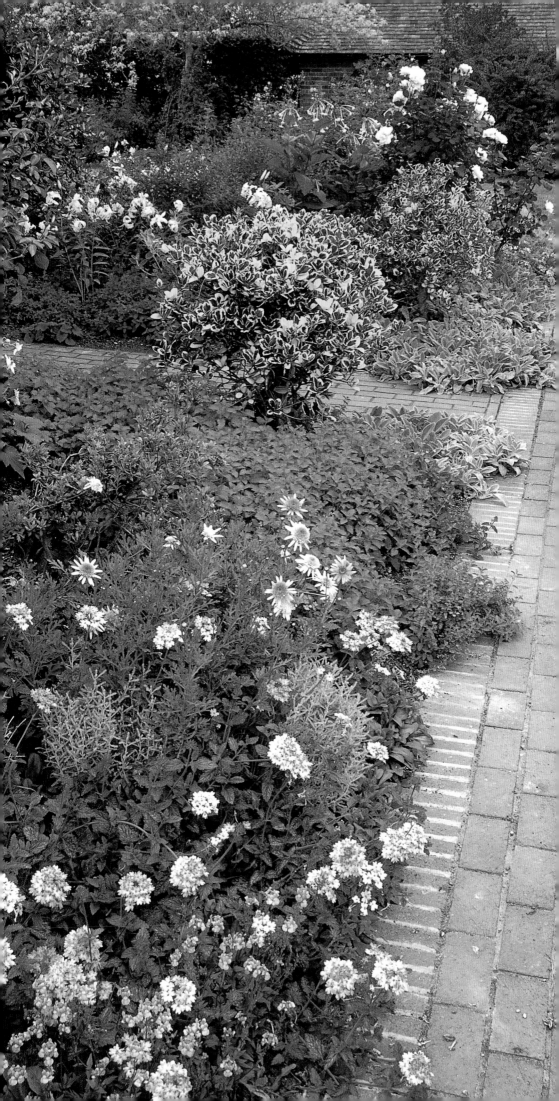

5 planting

Place the plants, still in their pots, in position, using the sand markings and/or the grid as a guide. Stand back, try to visualize them all fully grown, and adjust their positions accordingly. Start planting from the back of the plot and work toward the front edge. Set each plant to the same depth as it was in its pot. Firm in, water well, rake out the footprints, and then cover the bed with mulch.

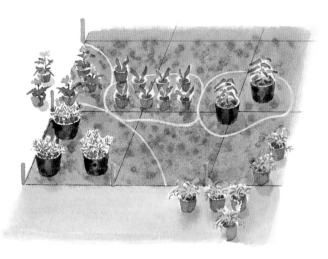

6 the mature plot

It will take two or more years for some of the plants—especially the shrubs—to fill out. Gaps can be filled with annuals, but there are unlikely to be enough mature plants in the first season to make a good display.

plant list

1 *Berberis thunbergii atropurpurea* x 2
2 *Rosa* 'Margaret Merril' x 2
3 *Buddleia* 'Lochinch' x 2
4 *Ilex aquifolium* 'Silver Queen' x 2
5 *Stachys lanata* x 6
6 *Nepeta faassenii* x 10
7 *Argyranthemum* 'Mary Wootton' x 4
8 *Verbena* 'Silver Anne' x 6
9 *Santolina pinnata neapolitana*
10 *Anemone* x *hybrida* 'Honorine Jobert' x 4
11 *Nicotiana sylvestris* x 6
12 *Lilium speciosum album* x 6
13 *Dianthus* 'Doris' x 12
14 *Phlox* 'Silver Salmon' x 4
15 *Convallaria majalis* x 16
16 *Lavandula angustifolia* x 6
17 *Matthiola incana* x 12
18 *Pelargonium* 'Sweet Mimosa' x 10
19 *Nicotiana* 'Evening Fragrance' x 24
20 *Aster pilosus demotus* x 4

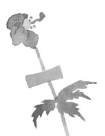

7 maintenance

Keep the beds tidy, removing flower heads once they begin to fade. In autumn, and again in spring, top-dress between the plants with organic matter, such as farmyard manure.

1 drawing up the plan

When laying out a new border, first draw up a plan on graph paper. Try to avoid conflicting colors and fragrances, and balance flowering throughout the season. It helps to use different colors to mark out positions of annuals and bedding plants (red), perennials (blue), and trees and shrubs (green).

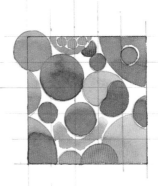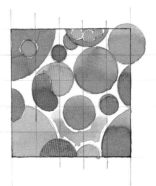

2 ground preparation

Prepare the ground in autumn for spring planting. This allows time for the soil to break down; also, any residual perennial weeds will reappear and can be removed. While digging, add as much organic material as possible; it will be some years before the border is dug again.

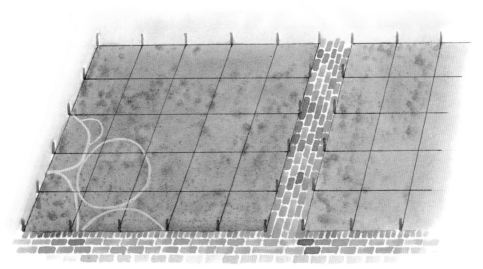

3 collecting the plants

It takes a while to gather together the plants for a large border. Some will have to be bought from nurseries and others will need propagating. Start in plenty of time or you may have to leave gaps in the border to be planted later. Try to collect the plants in the previous year; keep them in their pots in a cold frame until they are required.

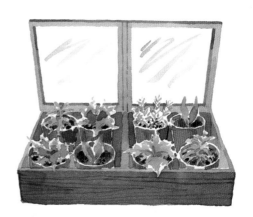

4 marking out the ground

Copy your sketched planting plan onto the ground using light-colored sand to mark the outline of each individual group of plants. To make this easier, lay out a grid of strings held in position by pegs, which corresponds to the grid drawn on your graph paper plan.

19

day and night scented border

Some paths in a garden are used regularly, and there is every reason to edge such busy thoroughfares with flower borders that produce rich scents from early in the morning right through to late evening. This is perfectly possible because some plants release their scent to attract daytime pollinators, while others that rely on night-flying moths and other insects are at their sweetest from dusk onward. Areas adjacent to open windows are also good locations for such borders, because the house is always filled with perfume.

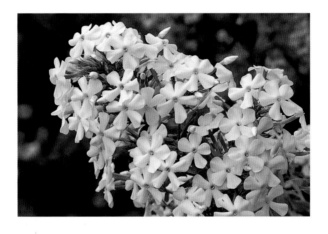

materials & equipment

20 ft (6 m) of wooden trellis
2 x 2 in (5 x 5 cm) wooden battens
wall plugs
galvanized screws and nails

spade
shovel
fork
rake
pruning shears
trowel
pegs and string
light-colored sand and bottle

plants in variety
well-rotted organic material

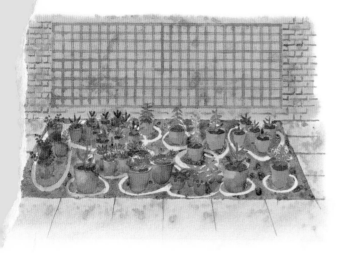

5 checking appearance

Before planting, stand the plants, still in their pots, in position. Try to visualize how the border will look when mature and make any adjustments that might seem necessary. Plant starting from the back so that you can easily see the plants' relation to one another as you work.

6 maintenance

Several of the plants are annuals—or perennials treated as annuals—and will need to be replaced every year. They can be purchased either as young plants or as seed. When buying plants, check the label carefully—not all varieties are scented. Plants can be held in large pots until after the frosts have passed.

plant list

1 *Nicotiana alata* 'Evening Fragrance' x 5
2 *Rosmarinus officinalis* x 1
3 *Oenothera biennis* x 1
4 *Rosa* 'Chianti' x 1
5 *Phlox* 'Europa' x 1
6 *Phlox paniculata alba* x 1
7 *Helitropium arborescens* 'Marine' x 6
8 *Dianthus* 'Mrs Sinkins' x 6
9 *Lavandula angustifolia* x 2
10 *Cestrum parqui* x 1
11 *Nicotiana alata* 'Fragrant Cloud' x 10
12 *Rosa* 'Jayne Austin' x 1
13 *Nepeta racemosa* x 4
14 *Lonicera periclymenum* x 1
15 *Jasminum officinale* x 4

pruning the lavender

Lavender needs an annual shearing if it is to be kept neat and compact. In autumn, remove all flower stems. During the following spring cut back the previous year's growth almost to where it starts (it is the lighter-colored wood).

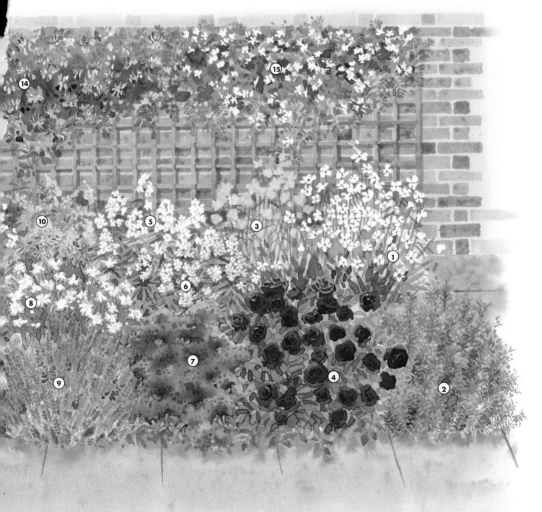

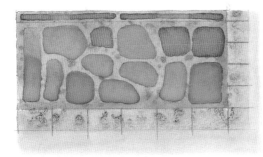

1 mapping the scents

The plot here measures 8 x 20 ft (2.5 x 6 m); before starting to plant, it is a good idea to sketch out a plan on paper. There are no strict rules as to where you should position the plants, but be mindful of segregating perfumes; it helps to mark day scented, evening scented, and touch scented plants on your drawn plan using different colors (here green, red, and blue respectively).

2 preparing the border

A scented border will generally do best in a warm, sunny aspect. A site backed by a wall is best, because this will give out stored heat after dark, enhancing the perfume of night-scented plants; it also allows scented climbers to be supported on a trellis. Prepare the ground thoroughly in the autumn; in spring, rake the ground through, removing any weeds that have reappeared.

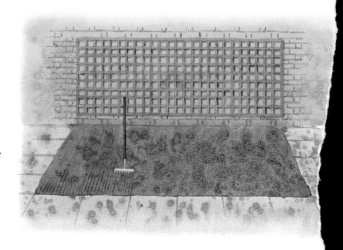

3 fixing the trellis

Perfumed climbing plants can be planted against a wall on a trellis. Fix the trellis panels by first attaching battens to the wall and then fixing the trellis to them. This provides space for the plants to twine behind the bars of the trellis.

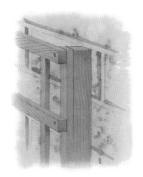

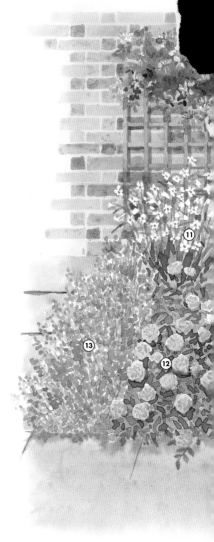

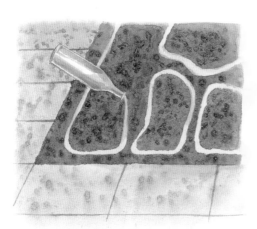

4 marking out the plan

Mark out the area that each plant will occupy when mature. Use light-colored sand poured onto the soil from a bottle. Alternatively mark out the plot by drawing a stick through the soil. This will help you avoid planting too tightly.

scented knot garden

Knot gardens are among the earliest forms of decorative planting, and they still hold much attraction for modern designers. Although the hedged patterns have a distinctly medieval feel about them, they also have a graphic quality that appeals to today's garden owners, especially if the hedging is scented. Once created, knot gardens are long-lived features and, although their structure remains the same from one year to the next, their contents and colors can change with the seasons and with the years.

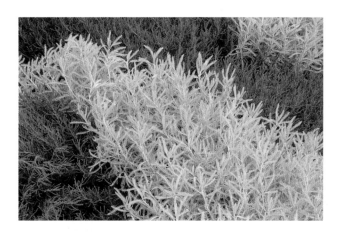

materials & equipment

5 plant stakes, 3 ft (90 cm) long
5 tree ties
sand (on heavy soils)

spade
fork
rake
pegs and string
trowel
shears

plants in variety
well-rotted organic material

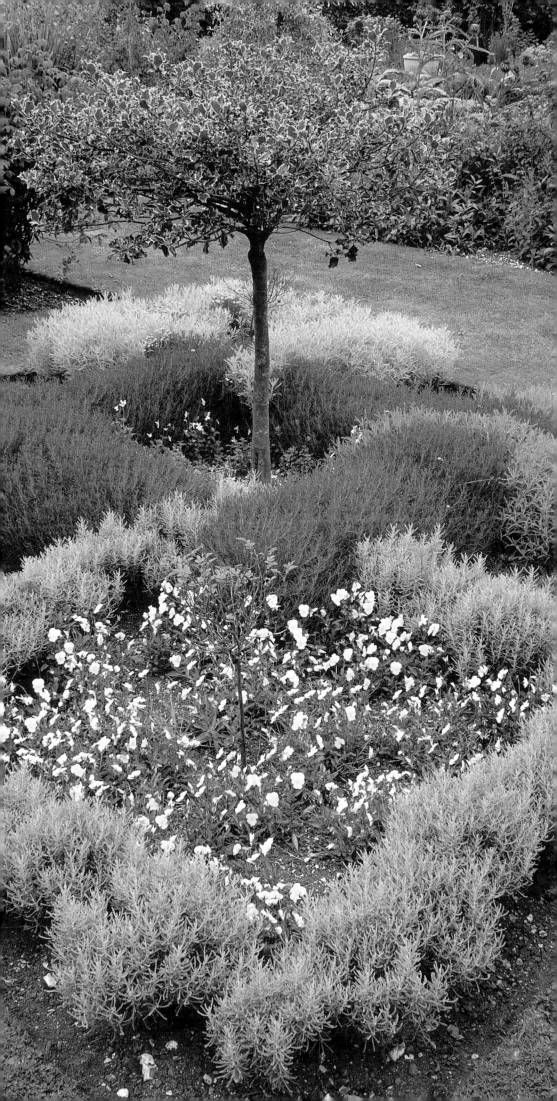

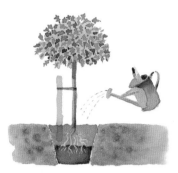

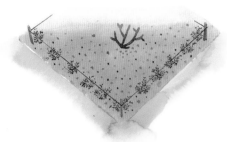

5 planting the holly tree

Plant the central holly tree (*Ilex aquifolium*) before setting out the hedges to avoid damaging the santolina. In spring, dig a large hole and work compost into the base. Spread out the roots, refill, and water. Secure the tree to a stake using a tree tie about 12 in (30 cm) above ground.

6 planting the roses and hedges

Plant the roses before setting out the hedge; you can use bushes or half-standards—the latter will need to be staked in the same manner as the holly standard. Plant the santolina at 12 in (30 cm) intervals using the strings as a guide. Water well. If the garden is in an exposed position, put up a temporary windbreak of plastic netting until the plants are established. Once established the santolina is quite tough and will even withstand sea-breezes.

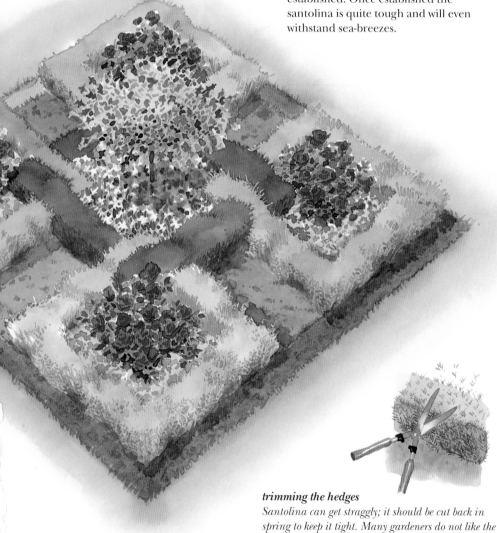

trimming the hedges

Santolina can get straggly; it should be cut back in spring to keep it tight. Many gardeners do not like the combination of its yellow flowers and silver foliage and remove the flower buds before they open.

7 mature knot garden

The knot garden will seem full of holes when first planted, but the santolina will soon fill out into a thick hedge. The hedges will look their best if kept neatly trimmed. Always remove dead and dying plants from the fill-in planting—an empty square looks better than one with messy vegetation.

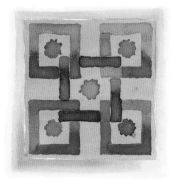

1 planning the garden

Knot gardens need very careful planning to get the scale and proportions right. For this reason, it is best to work out the design on graph paper before planting even a small garden, such as this 13 x 13 ft (4 x 4 m) plot. The design can come from your own head or be copied from an historic garden. The pattern can be geometric or include curved flowing lines, such as in those used in paisley designs. The simplest designs are often the most effective; more complicated patterns are best seen from above—from an upstairs window, for example.

2 preparing the ground

Because the garden will be in place for a long time, it is important to prepare the ground thoroughly. Remove or kill every piece of perennial weed and dig in plenty of well-rotted organic matter. Santolina, which makes up the hedges, likes a free-draining soil so dig in sand to improve drainage if necessary.

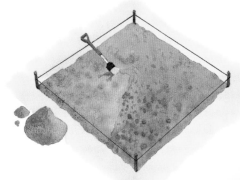

3 marking out

Mark out the position of the santolina hedges using pegs and string. If your design involves curves, first draw a grid over your plan, then lay out a similar grid on the ground with pegs and string. Using the grid as a guide, draw the curves on the ground using a bottle filled with dry sand as a marker.

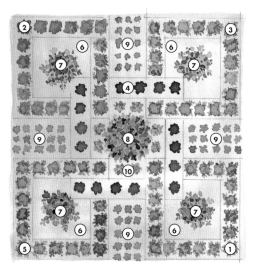

4 planting scheme

The planting within the hedged areas is a mixture of tall perennials surrounded by an ever-changing scene of annuals. Here, roses are underplanted with violas in the four outer squares, nicotiana surrounds a holly standard in the middle square, and chamomile lawns fill the open squares.

plant list
1 *Santolina chamaecyparissus* 'Lambrook Silver' x 19
2 *S. pinnata neapolitana* x 19
3 *S. pinnata neapolitana* 'Sulphurea' x 19
4 *S. rosmarinifolia* x 16
5 *S. chamaecyparissus nana* x 19
6 *Viola* 'Jeannie Bellew' x 100
7 *Rosa* 'Fragrant cloud' (half standard) x 4
8 *Ilex aquifolium* 'Silver Queen' (standard) x 1
9 *Chamaemelum nobile* 'Treneague' x 60
10 *Nicotiana* 'Domino White' x 8

herb garden

The idea of a herb garden immediately conjures up images of soft colors, heady fragrances, and the humming of bees. Well planned and thoughtfully planted, it can indeed be the height of sensual pleasure. As well as being decorative and fragrant, the garden will also provide a steady supply of fresh and dried herbs for the kitchen. Herb gardens need a good deal of maintenance to keep them tidy and productive, but the atmosphere they create is well worth the effort.

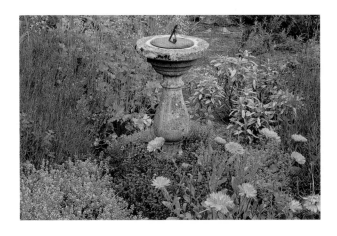

materials & equipment

2 paving slabs, 18 x 18 in (45 x 45 cm), per 3 ft (90 cm) of path
12 paving bricks per 3 ft (90 cm) of path
2 stone ornaments

spade
fork
rake
trowel
tamper or garden roller
pegs and string

herbs in variety
well-rotted organic material

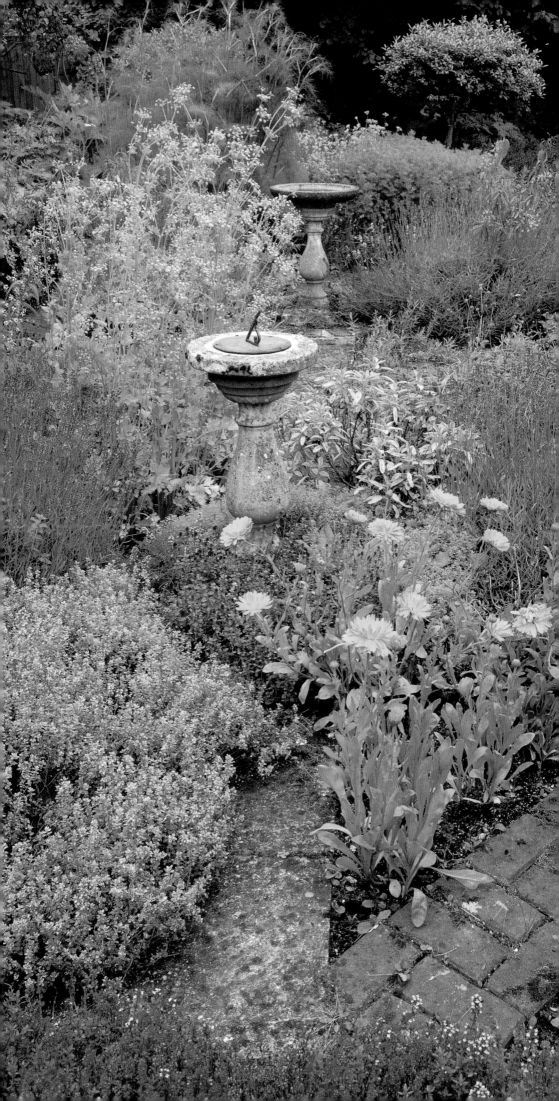

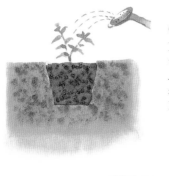

6 planting

In spring, set the pots in position on the prepared ground and then stand back and try to visualize the plants in full growth. Adjust their positions if necessary. Plant the herbs in the ground at the same depth as they were in their containers. Firm them in, level the soil, and water well.

7 the mature bed

The completed bed will soon fill out. Keep it well watered in dry weather and cut back herbaceous plants as they begin to fade in order to encourage new growth. In the autumn, cut out all dead and dying material. Prune back the shrubs if necessary—they should be kept reasonably compact.

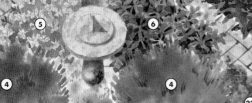

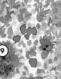
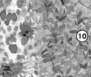
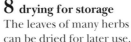

plant list

1 *Thymus* x *citriodorus* 'Nyewoods'
2 *Thymus serpyllum*
3 *Thymus vulgaris*
4 *Lavandula angustifolia*
5 *Coriandrum sativum*
6 *Salvia officinalis*
7 *Ocimum basilicum* 'Purpurascens'
8 *Sanguisorba minor*
9 *Rosmarinus officinalis*
10 *Mentha* x *villosa alopecuroides*
11 *Artemisia dracunculus*
12 *Origanum vulgare* 'Aureum'
13 *Aloysia triphylla*
14 *Mentha spicata*
15 *Levisticum officinale*
16 *Borago officinalis*
17 *Foeniculum vulgare*
18 *Allium schoenoprasum*
19 *Melissa officinalis*
20 *Helichrysum angustifolium*
21 *Calendula officinalis*
22 *Petroselinum crispum*
23 *Mentha suaveolens* 'Variegata'

8 drying for storage

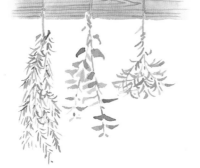

The leaves of many herbs can be dried for later use. Pick whole stems of young leaves, preferably before the plant comes into flower. Hang them upside down in small bunches in a warm, airy place. Once the leaves have dried, remove them from the stalks and store in an air-tight container.

1 designing the beds and paths

Carefully draw out the shape of the beds and hard landscaping on paper before starting work. Keep the pattern simple for ease of construction. The plot shown here measures 13 x 13 ft (4 x 4 m) and includes sufficient runs of paving to allow all the plants to be reached without having to walk over the soil. You can also add the layout of the plants to your plan if you wish.

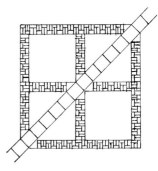

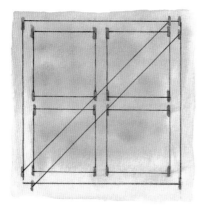

2 marking out

Lay out the plan on the ground using pegs and strings to mark the line of the paths. To ensure that all the right angles are true, measure the distance across the diagonals. If they are not the same, adjust the alignment of the strings until they are. The beds should then be perfectly square.

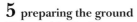

3 laying the paths

Because the paths will not take heavy traffic, just casual wandering among the herbs for maintenance and harvesting, they can be laid directly onto the soil without any foundations. If the soil is crumbly, simply ram it down with a tamper, rake over the surface to level it, and then lay the slabs and bricks. For a heavier soil, apply a 1 in (2 cm) layer of sand to bed in the slabs and bricks.

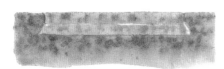

4 brick patterns

Bricks can be laid in a variety of patterns. For the 15 in (38 cm) wide path shown here, they can be laid in three parallel rows, or alternated, with two across and one upright followed by one upright and two across. For wider paths there are many more permutations of pattern.

5 preparing the ground

Thoroughly dig the ground in the autumn, removing all perennial weeds. Because the herbs will be in place for many years, it is vital to begin with a weed-free plot. Dig in plenty of well-rotted organic material, such as manure or compost, before planting in spring.

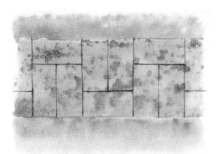

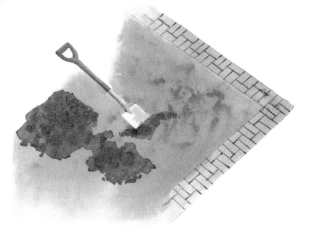

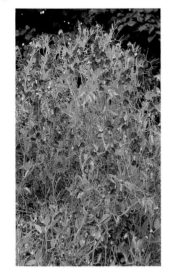

climbing plants

Scented climbers have an incredibly romantic image. One only has to think of honeysuckle, roses, jasmine, and wisteria to conjure up images of relaxing in sweet-smelling arbors, or opening windows to let in the perfumes of plants on outside walls. Climbers are fairly easy to maintain; they provide a vertical element in the garden and are ideal for barriers and screens. It is difficult to imagine a garden without them.

above The sweet pea is one of the most important annual scented climbers. It comes in a wide range of soft and bright colors. It makes an excellent cut flower to perfume the house as well as the garden.

right Roses are the quintessential scented climber, especially when they are as prolific as this *Rosa brunonii* 'La Mortola'.

below Rambling roses can weave together colors and textures in the garden.

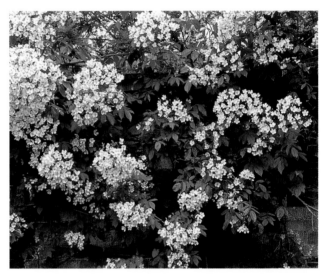

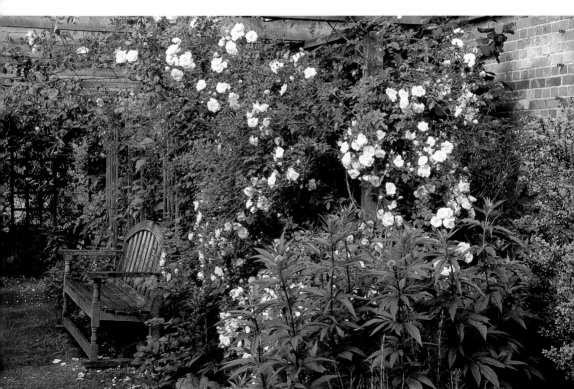

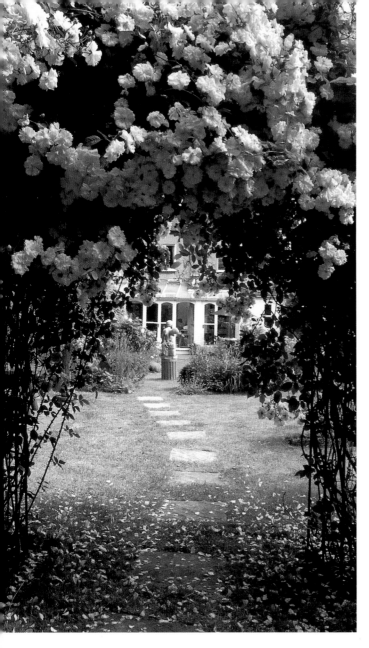

left Archways link different areas of the garden. They show a glimpse of what lies beyond, drawing the viewer closer and eventually through. Their impact is enhanced by scented flowers. Here the fragrant *Rosa* 'Adélaïde d'Orléans' creates a beautiful frame.

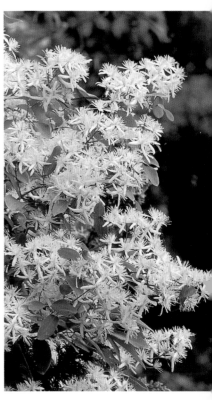

above Clematis is a very versatile plant, suited to most climates and aspects. Most of the large, colorful varieties are not scented, but many of the smaller ones make up for their lack of size and color with a strong perfume and profuse blooms. This prodigious flowerer is the highly scented *Clematis paniculata*.

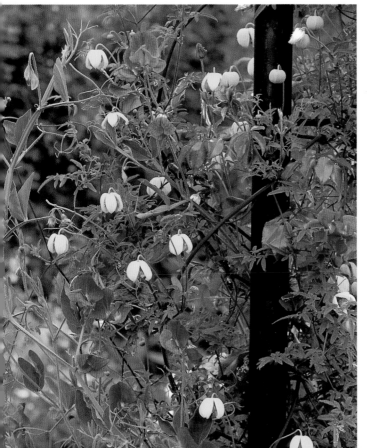

left Sweet peas are spectacular scented annuals that can be trained up supports or grown among shrubs. Although their flowering period is long, they begin to dwindle by the end of the summer. It is a good idea to grow them with other colorful climbers that flower later. Here they are with the unscented *Clematis orientalis*.

honeysuckle porch

One of the most romantic smells must be that of honeysuckle. This is a scent evocative of country lanes, cottage gardens, and romantic trysts. It is particularly pleasing during the evening, especially as dusk falls. There are a variety of places it can be grown in the garden, but possibly the best is over a gazebo where you might sit relaxing as the light fades, or over a house porch, so that the scent wafts in through the open door on the evening breeze.

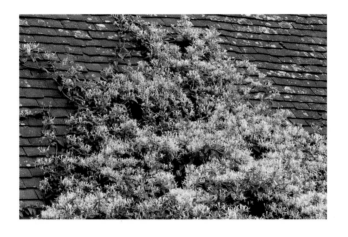

materials & equipment

bamboo canes
galvanized wire
eye bolts
wall plugs
plant ties
chipped bark mulch

drill
hammer
pliers
wire cutters
spade
pruning shears

2 *Lonicera similis delavayi* plants
well-rotted organic material

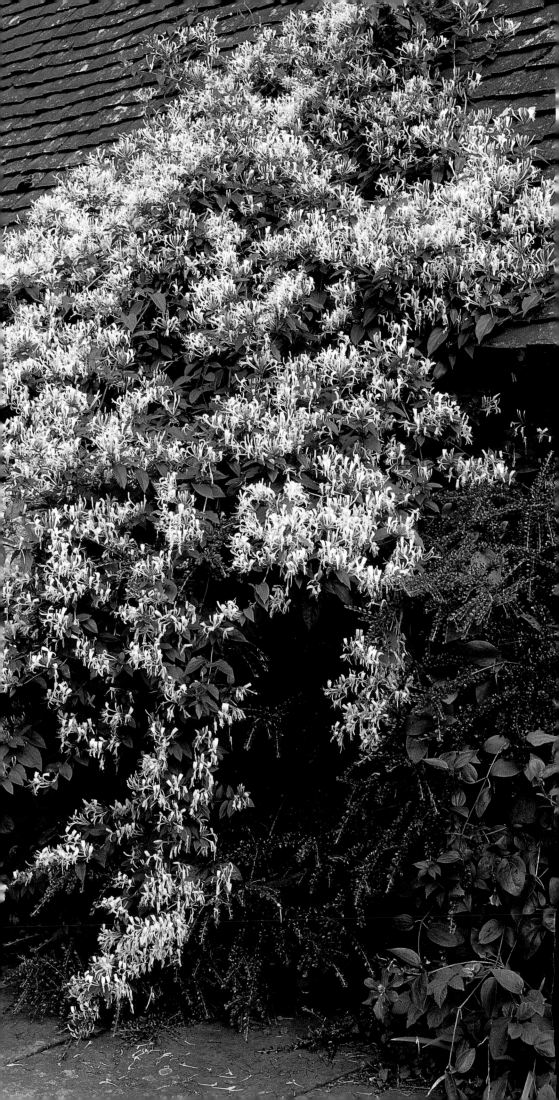

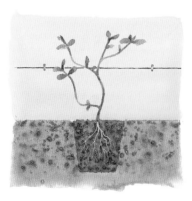
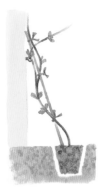

5 planting the honeysuckle

Plant one honeysuckle bush on either side of the structure. Dig the planting holes at least 12 in (30 cm) away from the walls. Plant so that the top of the rootball is level with the soil surface. Water well and mulch with chipped bark.

6 initial training

Lead the stems toward the wire supports using canes tipped at an angle from the rootball to the wall. Avoid damaging the roots as you push the canes into the ground. Tie the stems to the cane and, when larger, directly to the wires.

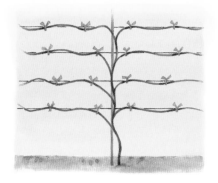

7 covering the wall

Fan out the shoots to cover all the wires. Spread out the shoots at the base of the wall; similarly spread out any side shoots that emerge further up the plant to cover the entire wall. Tie in the shoots with string or plant ties.

8 care and maintenance

Honeysuckle need not be pruned at all, but removing dead material helps prevent a build-up of weight as well as making the plant look fresher and neater.

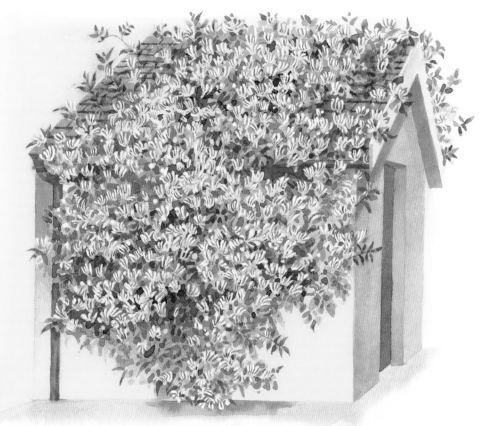

1 location

Many houses have a side or front porch or an attached building, such as a garage or shed. These are often later additions to the house that add little to its original character. Covering the building with honeysuckle, roses, jasmine, or wisteria will help disguise its appearance and fill the house with scent. Even attractive porches can be enhanced by having honeysuckle growing round them.

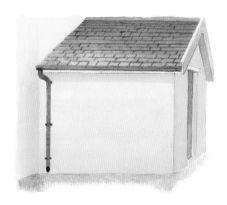

2 the wall supports

Climbing plants such as honeysuckle are best supported by horizontal galvanized wires, firmly anchored to the wall at 18 in (45 cm) intervals. Each wire is secured at its ends by eye bolts screwed or hammered into the wall (see page 45). Bend the wire back on itself, twisting it around with pliers to keep it as taut as possible. The wires and eye bolts can be painted the same color as the wall to make them less visible.

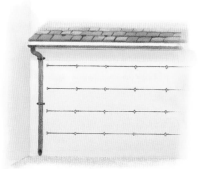

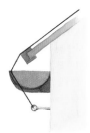

3 roof supports

Honeysuckle will clamber over a roof on its own, but wire supports will give it a better grip in strong winds, especially while it is becoming established. Screw vine eyes into the facial boards on either side of the roof at 8 in (45 cm) intervals and draw the wire taut over the roof.

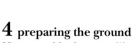

protecting the tiles

Use treated wooden spacing blocks to lift the wires off the roof shingles. This gives the honeysuckle more space in which to twine around the wire and protects the shingles from damage. The blocks are made by simply nailing together three pieces of wood in a "sandwich." The middle piece should be just a little thicker than a shingle, and should be slightly recessed, so that the whole assembly can be slipped over the edges of the shingles.

4 preparing the ground

Honeysuckle does not like to be dry at the roots, so add a generous amount of organic material to the soil at the base of the wall. This fibrous material holds plenty of moisture but allows excess rain to drain away. While digging, make sure that all perennial weeds are removed.

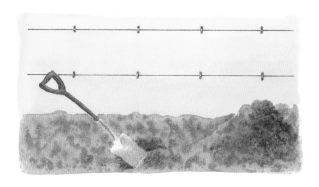

sweet pea obelisk

The distinctive scent of sweet peas seems to be loved by everyone, probably because it is particularly evocative of childhood. Sweet peas are not just for decorating and perfuming the garden; they make excellent cut flowers for taking into the house or giving to friends and visitors. They are easy to grow and can be used in many decorative ways in the garden, from growing up tripods to allowing them to scramble through shrubs with gay abandon.

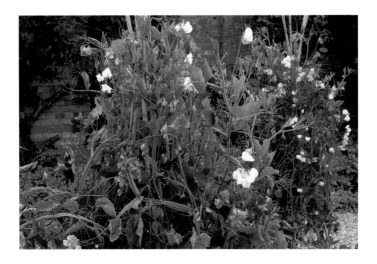

materials & equipment

4 canes or poles, 8 ft (2.5 m) long
garden string

spade
trowel
knife

sweet pea seed, *Lathyrus odoratus*
well-rotted organic material

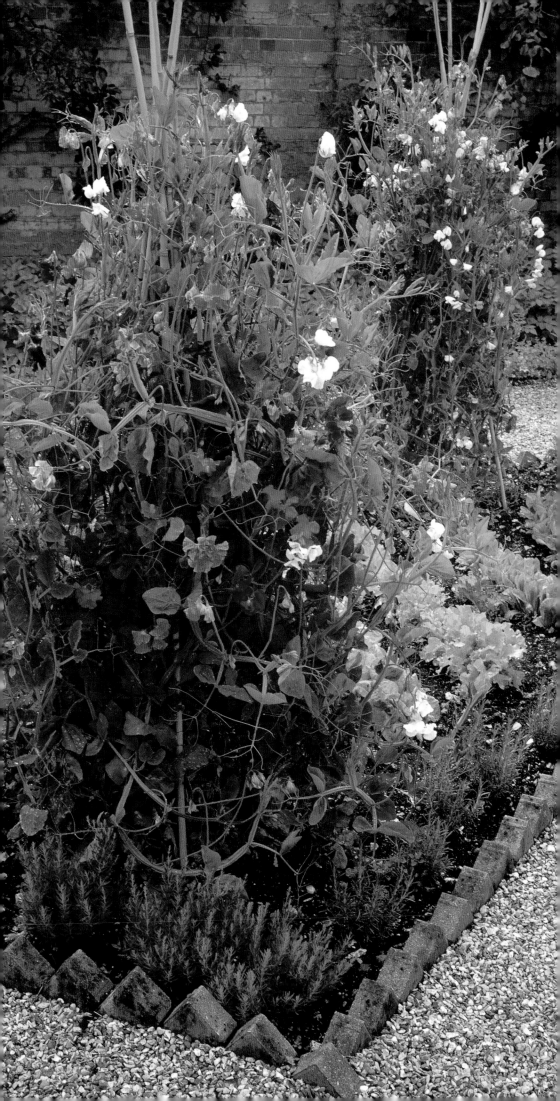

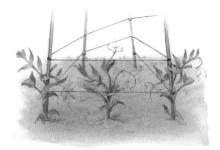

5 planting

Plant the peas at 8 in (20 cm) intervals around the base of the obelisk. The peas will need to be tied to the canes or string to start with, but will soon be self-supporting. Handle the young stems carefully because they may be brittle at this stage. It is wise to put down slug pellets after planting; slugs will eat right through the succulent young pea stems.

6 in full flower

Sweet peas flower from the summer to early autumn. Old fashioned varieties produce small but highly scented flowers in blues, reds, pinks, and whites. Newer cultivars are available in almost all colors; and because they produce larger flowers, they may be more suitable for cutting. Do not let flowers on the plant run to seed—cut them off as they fade.

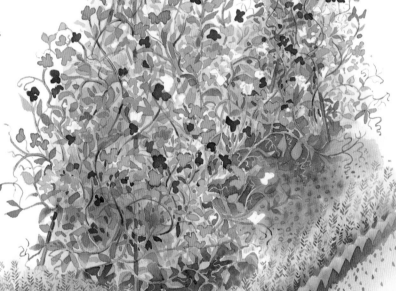

alternative supports

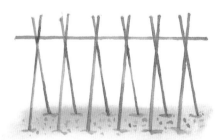

sweet pea wall

Sweet peas do not have to be trained up an obelisk; a "wall" of sweet peas can be made by arranging canes as above. Alternatively, sweet peas can be grown up trellising, wire rings, or through shrubs that have flowered in the spring.

container planting

Sweet peas can be grown successfully in containers. They do best in large pots and should be supported with sticks or a tepee of poles. Water the container at least once a day, and twice or more on hot, dry days; apply liquid feed every two weeks. Again, the plants should be dead-headed to encourage flowering.

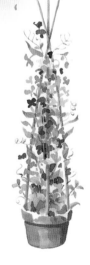

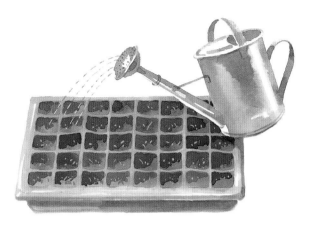

1 sowing

In early spring, sow sweet pea seeds into a good compost in cellular trays. If you use fibrous trays, the resulting seedlings can be planted out without disturbing the roots. Sow one seed per cell, water, and leave in a warm place, out of direct sunlight. Sweet peas can also be bought as seedlings, although there is a much greater choice of colors and scents when grown from seed.

2 pinching out the tips

When the seedlings have reached 4 in (10 cm), pinch out the tops of the stem just above the nearest set of leaves. If you buy the plants as seedlings, avoid lanky and overcrowded specimens, and look carefully for any evidence of pests and disease.

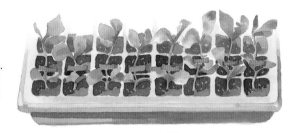

3 making the frame

Prepare the ground thoroughly, removing any weeds and adding plenty of organic material to rejuvenate the soil. Push four canes into the ground (or more for a bigger structure), about 16 in (40 cm) apart, so that their tops meet to form a pyramid. Make certain that each cane is firmly anchored. Tie their tops together in the manner of a tepee.

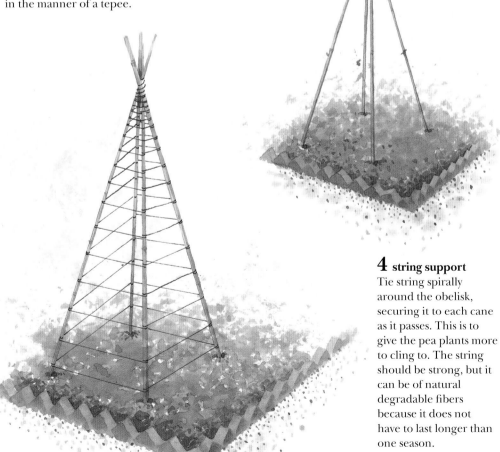

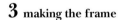

4 string support

Tie string spirally around the obelisk, securing it to each cane as it passes. This is to give the pea plants more to cling to. The string should be strong, but it can be of natural degradable fibers because it does not have to last longer than one season.

scented wall

One way of really enjoying plants is to grow them up walls. Not only does this perfume the area below the plant—perhaps a patio where you sit—but also the house itself. Open windows and doors invite the scent to waft in. How relaxing to fall asleep with the fragrance of honeysuckle, wisteria, or roses filling the bedroom. Another advantage of this planting is that walls usually retain the day's heat, and this warmth helps the plants to release their scent.

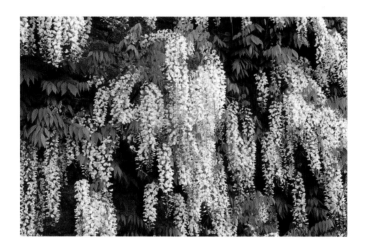

materials & equipment

6 ft (2 m) cane
plant ties
eye bolts
wall plugs
turnbuckle
galvanized wire

spade
pruning shears
masonry bits
hammer
pliers
drill

1 *Wisteria floribunda* 'Alba'
garden compost or soil conditioner

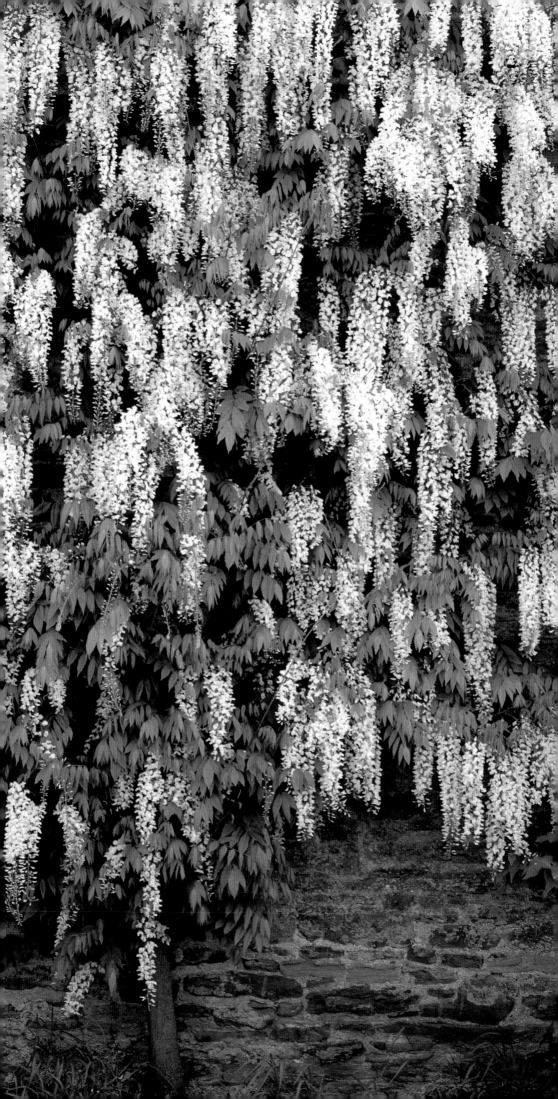

trellis and mesh as supports

Climbers can be supported on wooden trellising or plastic mesh as alternatives to taut wires. Trellis should be screwed to the wall using a spacing block of wood, so that the bars are not tight against the wall; or it can be fixed using hinges at the bottom and hooks at the top of the trellis panels. This allows the trellis panels to be eased away gently from the wall for painting and maintenance. Plastic mesh is fastened to the wall with special clips; again, these allow for removal if the wall needs to be repaired or decorated.

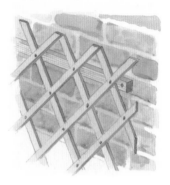

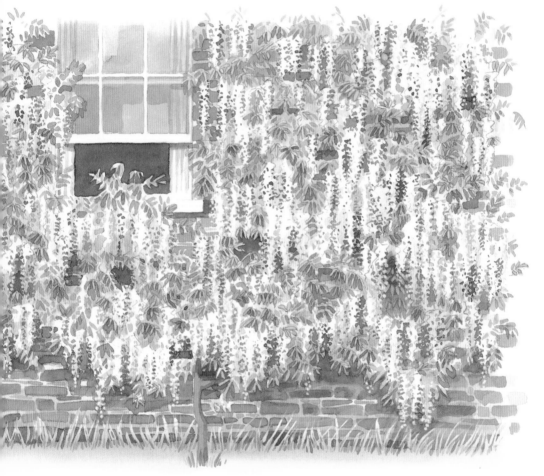

5 in flower

Wisteria floribunda 'Alba' produces dense clusters of pale, highly scented flowers in early summer. Even in winter, it is an attractive feature of any garden, its gnarled stem providing sculptural and textural interest.

6 pruning

Once it reaches the desired coverage, the wisteria needs regular pruning to keep it in check and maintain its flowering power. Immediately after flowering, cut back all the new growth to 6 in (15 cm) or four or five leaves. In the winter, reduce this further to 3–4 in (8–10 cm) or two to three buds.

1 wire supports

Climbing plants, including wisteria, can be supported discreetly on walls using wires stretched taut between eye bolts. The best flowers are produced in south-facing or part-shaded locations. Ensure the wall is in good repair—it will need to support quite a weight.

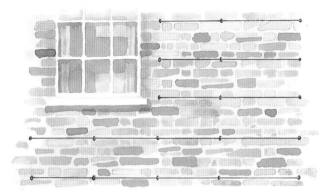

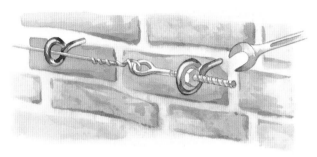

2 fixing the wires

The horizontal wires should be fixed 12–18 in (30–45 cm) apart and held in position with eye bolts at 32 in (80 cm) intervals. Drill holes at required positions, insert a wall plug, and screw in an eye bolt. Thread the wire through the eye bolts. Fasten the wire at one end using pliers to twist it back on itself. Use a turnbuckle at the other end to make the wire as taut as possible. Attach the bolt to the wall through an eye bolt.

eye bolts
These galvanized fasteners come in various shapes. Some are nailed into the wall; others screw into wall plugs.

3 planting

Work two buckets of organic material into the soil and plant the wisteria. It should be at least 12 in (30 cm) out from the base of the wall. Train the stem up to the first wires using a cane. Trim off any weak or broken shoots.

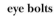

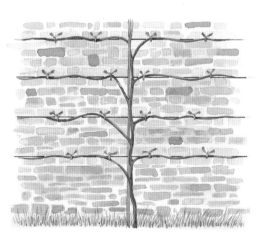

4 training

As the wisteria grows, train it horizontally along the wires, tying it in with string or plant ties. Other climbers can be used as alternatives. Honeysuckle (*Lonicera*) is an obvious choice, but choose carefully because not all are scented; the same applies to climbing roses. Another wonderfully scented climber is jasmine (*Jasminum officinale*).

rose growing through a tree

Scented climbers rambling up through old trees make a breathtaking sight and scent the air for some distance around. Some of the best climbers for this are the old rambling roses and honeysuckles. Many clematis species are also suitable, although the fragrant varieties tend to be those with small flowers, with the exception of the spring-flowering *Clematis montana*. Always choose a strong, sound tree; never use dead trees because these may break without warning.

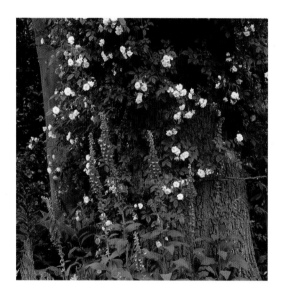

materials & equipment

sturdy rope
rubber padding
plant ties

spade
pruning shears

1 *Rosa* 'Félicité et Perpétue'
garden compost
chipped bark mulch

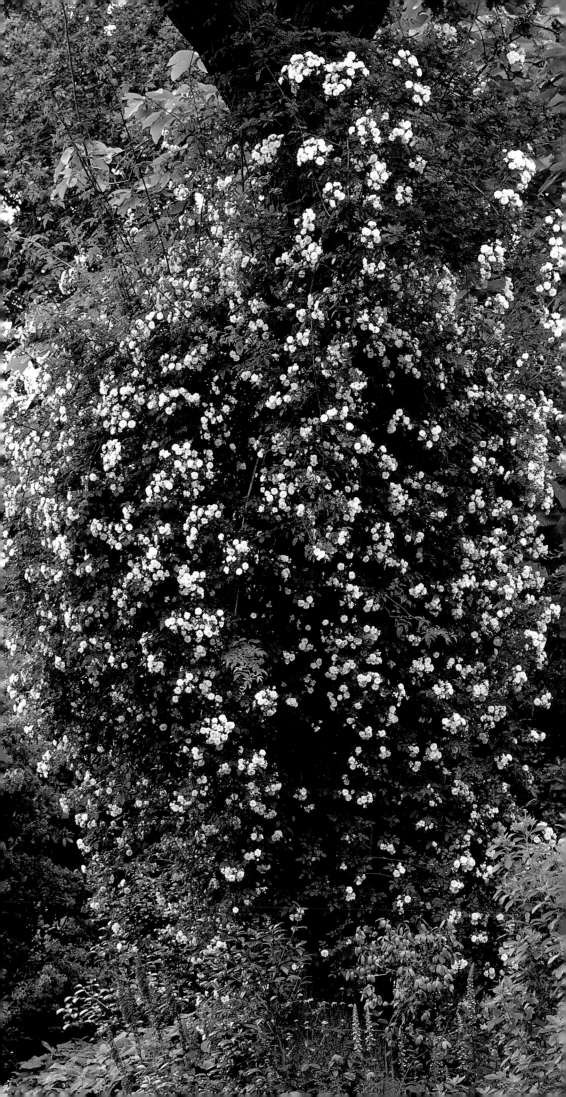

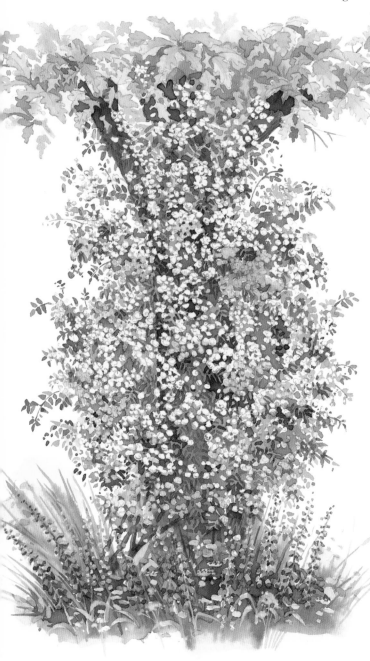

4 **the mature rose**
Eventually the rose will
reach up into the tree and
become self-supporting.
New shoots from the base
will grow up through the
increasing mass of stems,
and only the more
wayward will need tying
in. The rope can then be
detached or left in place if
it is causing the tree no
problem. It will take some
years before the tree is
completely covered—but
the wait is worthwhile.

alternative rose supports

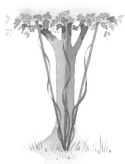

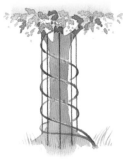

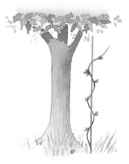

fan support
There are many other ways of
providing support for the rose (or
other climber) before it reaches the
lower tree branches. One way is to
push long canes into the ground
so that they extend from the rose
into the lower branches.

pole cage
A more attractive method is to
place canes all around the tree,
about 6 in (15 cm) or so from the
trunk, and train the rose shoots in
a spiral around the "cage." Use
hoops of wire to support the canes
and keep them equidistant.

visible trunk
To keep the trunk of the tree clear
so that it can be seen, grow the rose
up a single pole placed 2 ft
(60 cm) from the trunk. Whatever
support you use, never attach
anything constricting to the tree or
drive nails into its trunk.

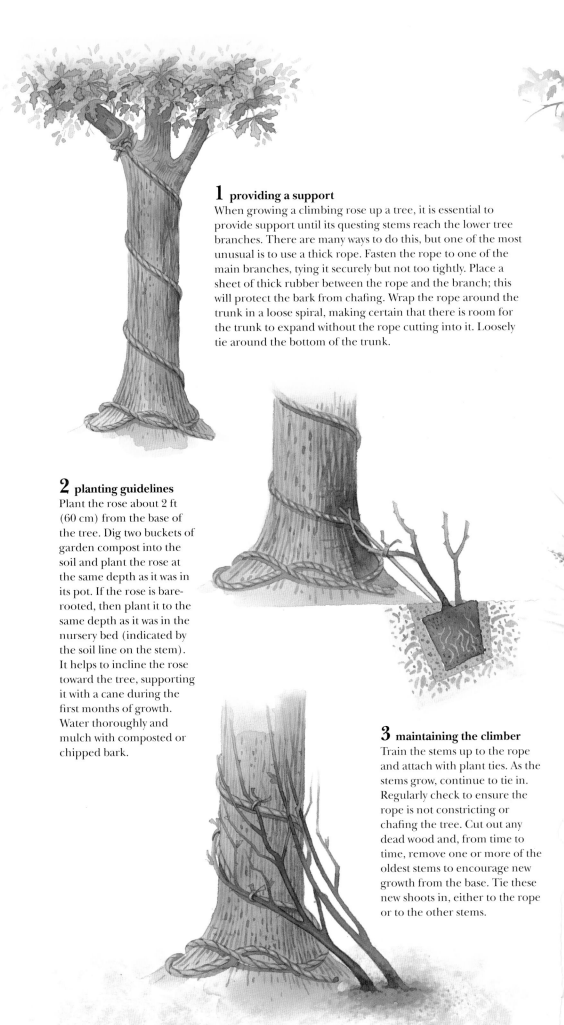

1 providing a support

When growing a climbing rose up a tree, it is essential to provide support until its questing stems reach the lower tree branches. There are many ways to do this, but one of the most unusual is to use a thick rope. Fasten the rope to one of the main branches, tying it securely but not too tightly. Place a sheet of thick rubber between the rope and the branch; this will protect the bark from chafing. Wrap the rope around the trunk in a loose spiral, making certain that there is room for the trunk to expand without the rope cutting into it. Loosely tie around the bottom of the trunk.

2 planting guidelines

Plant the rose about 2 ft (60 cm) from the base of the tree. Dig two buckets of garden compost into the soil and plant the rose at the same depth as it was in its pot. If the rose is bare-rooted, then plant it to the same depth as it was in the nursery bed (indicated by the soil line on the stem). It helps to incline the rose toward the tree, supporting it with a cane during the first months of growth. Water thoroughly and mulch with composted or chipped bark.

3 maintaining the climber

Train the stems up to the rope and attach with plant ties. As the stems grow, continue to tie in. Regularly check to ensure the rope is not constricting or chafing the tree. Cut out any dead wood and, from time to time, remove one or more of the oldest stems to encourage new growth from the base. Tie these new shoots in, either to the rope or to the other stems.

scented arbor

An arbor is the perfect place to sit and relax, especially after a day's work. The scent of the climbers that clothe the arbor and the nature of the structure itself combine to soothing effect. The arbor's leafy and flowery walls create a sense of safe enclosure without being boxed in; it is open and closed at the same time. Here a simple structure is covered with 'New Dawn', a repeat-flowering rose that continues to produce blooms all summer long.

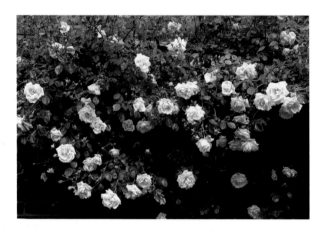

materials & equipment

2 wooden trellis panels 3 x 6 ft (90 cm x 1.8 m)
1 wooden trellis panel 6 x 8 ft (1.8 x 2.5 m)
1 wooden trellis panel 3 x 8 ft (90 cm x 2.5 m)
4 square wooden posts 4 in x 4 in x 8 ft (10 cm x 10 cm x 2.5 m)
4 wooden finials for posts
galvanized nails
2 buckets of stones
8 cu ft (0.25 m³) of concrete
plant ties
rustic bench

spade
shovel
hammer
level
saw
drill

2 *Rosa* 'New Dawn'
2 buckets of compost

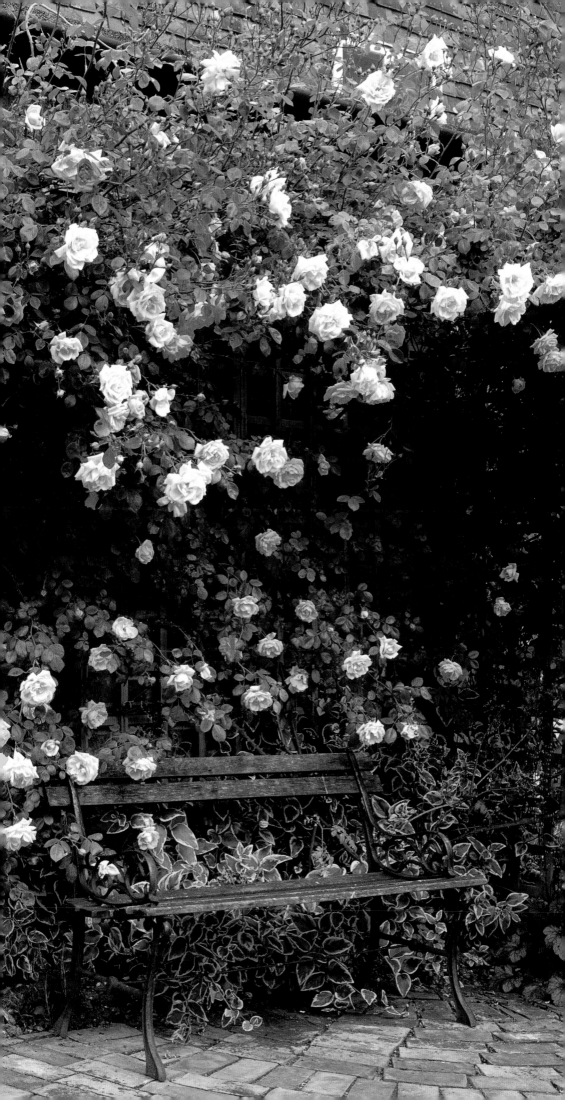

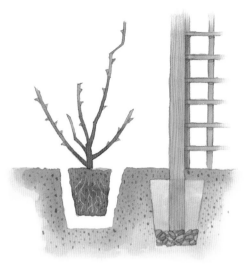

5 planting

Plant two roses, one at each of the back corners of the arbor. Prepare the ground by incorporating plenty of well-rotted organic material into the soil around the planting area. Dig a hole slightly wider than the rootball of the rose and then plant the rose so that the top of the rootball is level with top of the hole. Fill in with soil. Firm down the earth around the roots and water well.

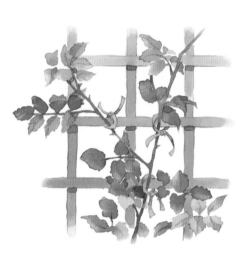

6 training the roses

Spread the stems of the newly-planted roses so that they fan out along the sides and back of the arbor. Tie in each shoot with string or a plant tie. As the shoots grow, continue to tie them in and arrange so that they eventually cover the whole arbor.

7 finished arbor

Like most climbing or rambling roses, *Rosa* 'New Dawn' is a vigorous plant that produces a profusion of blooms from mid-summer to autumn. It can even be grown successfully in partly shaded sites.

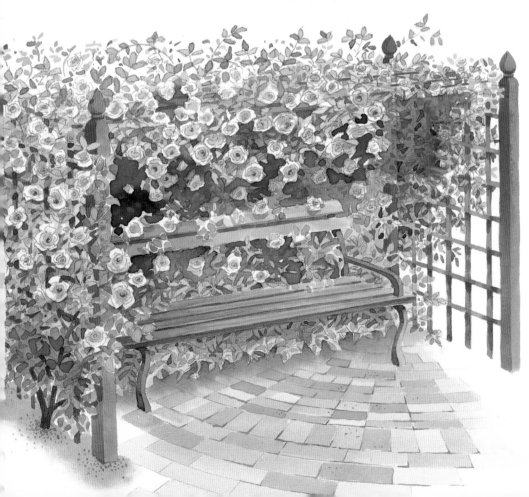

1 planning the arbor

Wooden or metal arbor frameworks are available ready-made in a variety of shapes and sizes. When buying the framework, allow ample space for table and chairs (if you plan to eat in the arbor) and for the spread of the rose, which will protrude at least 18 in (45 cm) into the seating area.

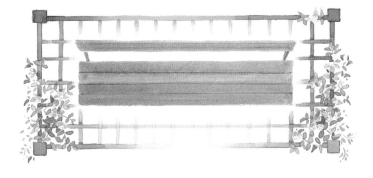

2 erecting the posts

If the arbor is in a sheltered place the posts can simply be buried in the ground 24 in (60 cm) deep and the earth rammed around them. For a more secure structure in an exposed position, the posts should be concreted in. Dig four holes 24 in (60 cm) deep and place 4 in (10 cm) of stones in the bottom. Use a level to ensure that that the posts are upright. Fill in the holes with concrete.

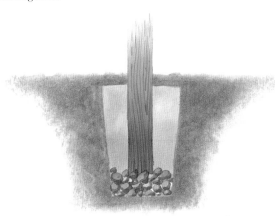

3 attaching the trellis

Fix the side and back trellis panels to the posts with galvanized nails. To prevent the wood splitting, drill pilot holes in the panels using an electric drill. Make certain that the panels are level. Nail or screw the decorative wooden finials to the four posts. Finials are available from mail order catalogs or nurseries in a wide variety of shapes.

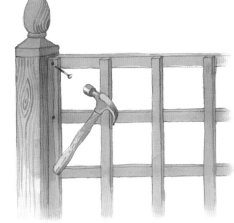

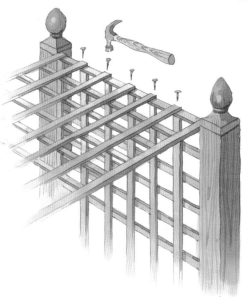

4 fixing the roof panel

Cut the roof panel so that it rests on both the side and back trellis panels. Attach the roof by nailing or screwing it directly to the side panels, drilling pilot holes first. If the top rails of the side panels are not strong enough to hold the weight of the roof, reinforce them with 1 x 2 in (2.5 x 5 cm) wooden battens along their length.

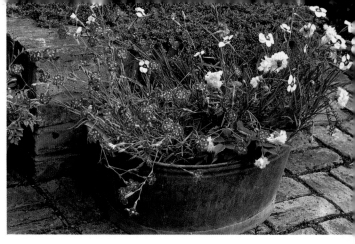

right A series of smaller pots of pinks (*Dianthus*) put into the larger container of a galvanized washtub forms an attractive group of scented plants. Using a large, unusual container in this way is a good method of dealing with plants in unattractive plastic pots.

container planting is a versatile

way of filling space and a great boon to any gardener, especially if space is at a premium. Even quite large pots are light enough to be moved, allowing a change of scene according to mood or season. Pots can be kept out of sight until they come into flower, and they let tender plants survive in temperate climates because they can be moved inside a greenhouse for the winter. Pots can also be used for temporary settings, such as placing evening-fragrant plants near a table for a dinner party.

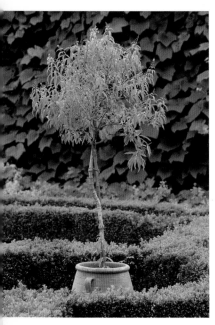

above Lemon verbena (*Aloysia triphylla*) has highly aromatic leaves, ideal for using in a potpourri and in the kitchen. Unfortunately, it is very delicate and must be wintered indoors to grow to a reasonable size.

right This simple but highly effective group of different-sized pots of spring-scented bulbs includes *Narcissus* 'Tête-à-tête', *Crocus chrysanthus* 'Snow Bunting', *Hyacinthus* 'Carnegie', and *H.* 'Blue Magic'.

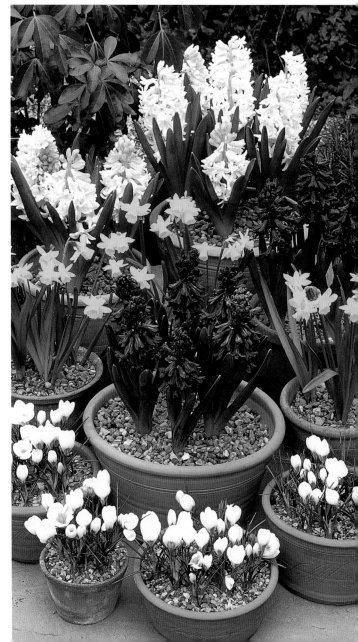

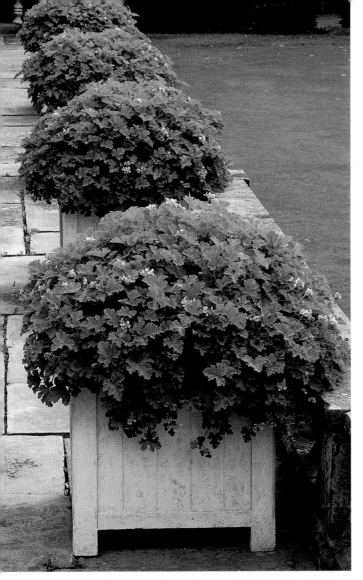

left Grouping containers can add formality to a garden. Here a regular arrangement of scented-leafed pelargoniums in white-painted Versailles tubs creates a very regular profile on the edge of a terrace.

below Good use can be made of a large container by filling it with different plants: here myrtle mixes with *Heliotropium* 'White Queen', *Hosta* 'Royal Standard', *Convolvulus cneorum*, *Pelargonium* 'Arctic Star', and *Osteospermum*.

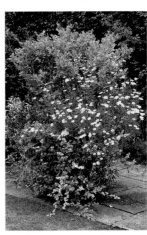

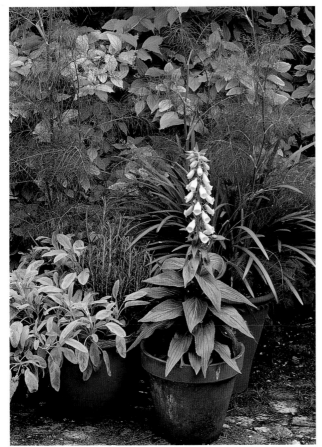

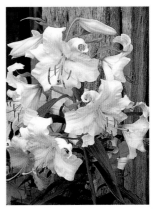

above Lilies are excellent container plants—many are highly scented and have a long flowering period. Positioning a pot by a doorway acts as a greeting to visitors and allows the scent to waft through the house.

left Herbs, such as fennel, sage, and rosemary, work well in containers but are not always very colorful. It is a good idea to mix in a few non-herbs, such as foxglove, for visual interest.

pelargoniums
in pots

Not all scents are immediately apparent to the nose. They do not hover in the air but need to be teased out of the plant by gently caressing the foliage. Such plants—which include scented pelargoniums, or scented-leaf geraniums—should be sited near a path so that their leaves are easily reached by passers-by. Another good position is next to a seat, so that anyone sitting there can idly crush a leaf to release its heady perfume. Planting pelargoniums in pots is particularly versatile because the plants can be moved around if the seats are relocated.

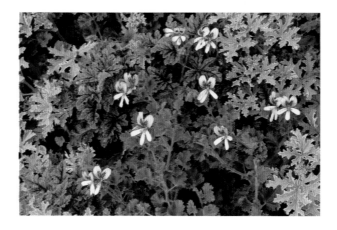

materials & equipment

5 terra-cotta pots
3 bricks
potting soil
broken pots for drainage
trowel

Pelargonium 'Royal Oak' x 1
P. 'Graveolens' x 2
P. 'Lady Plymouth' x 2

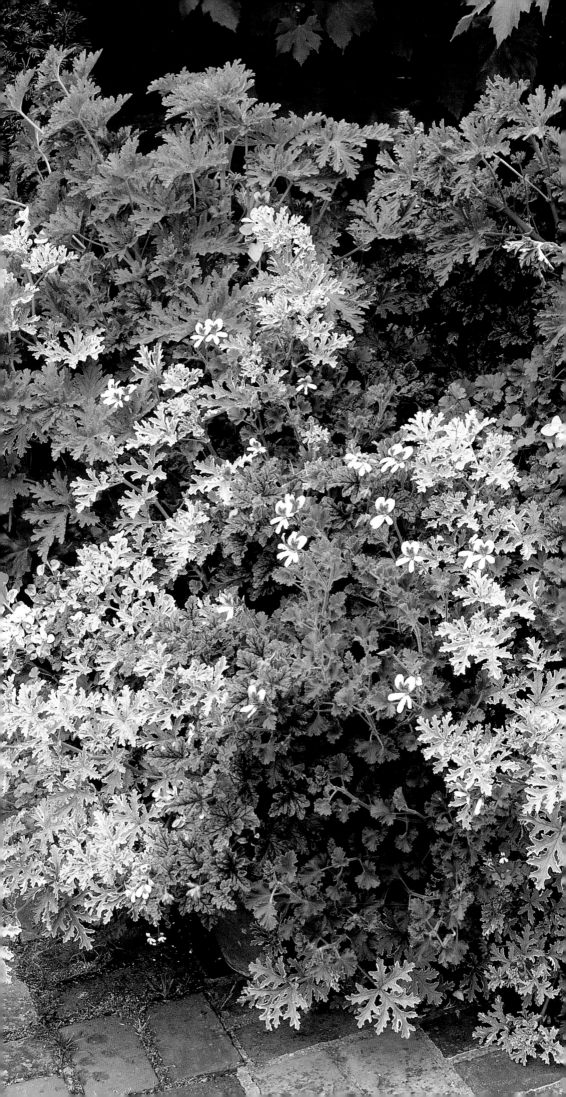

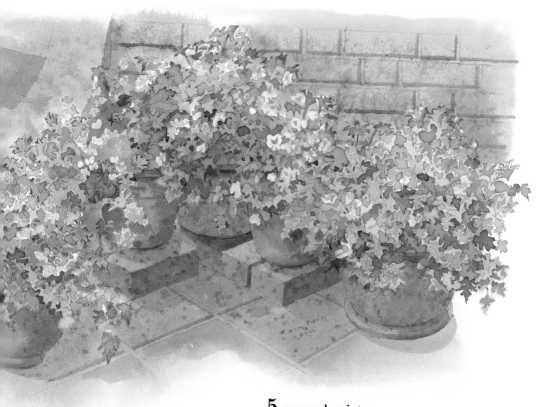

5 care and maintenance

Water the pots once a day. Even when it rains, pots near walls may receive little or no moisture, so check that they have enough. Feed with a liquid feed once every two weeks in the growing season.

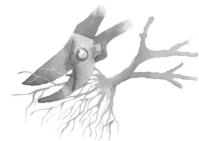

6 preparing for storage

The plants can be wintered over in their pots and cuttings taken in the spring. However, this is likely to take up a lot of space so it is better to take the plants out and place them all together in one container. First lift them out of their pots and shake gently so that much of the soil falls from their roots.

7 cutting back

Trim back the branches to about 4 in (10 cm) and remove any remaining leaves; trim back any straggling roots. Make the cuts as cleanly as possible—bruising may allow in infection.

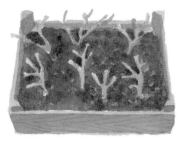

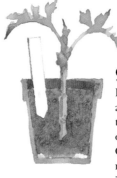

9 potting

Place the cuttings, six to a pot, in potting soil. Put the pots into plastic bags or a propagating tent. Once the cuttings have rooted, transplant them into individual pots. Keep under cover until they are established.

8 wintering over

Place the plants in a tray of just-moist soil. Keep over winter in a frost-free place, such as a garage. In spring, move them into the light to obtain new shoots for use as cutting material.

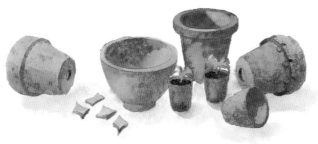

1 choosing pots

Virtually any container can be used, but pelargoniums seem to work best in conventional terra-cotta pots, which should be about 10 in (25 cm) wide. Larger pots can be used but should be planted in position as they will be heavy when filled.

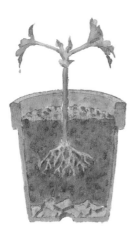

2 planting

When new plants are bought, they usually need to be transplanted into larger containers. Place broken pots or irregular stones over the hole in the bottom of a pot, and fill with enough potting soil so that the top of the rootball of the pelargonium is level with the surface. Fill with compost.

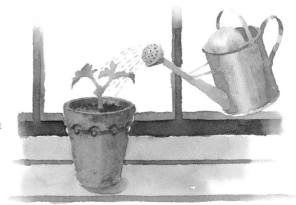

3 early care

Water the plants well. Keep in the greenhouse, solarium, or on a window sill until the threat of frost has passed. When first planted, they should be kept out of direct sunlight; drafts must be avoided.

4 siting the pots

Choose a warm position, preferably against a wall. The warmth will help to bring out the scent of the pelargoniums. The pots will look dull if all on the same level. Place the back ones on bricks or upturned pots so that a more effective display is created. This will also give all the plants good access to available light.

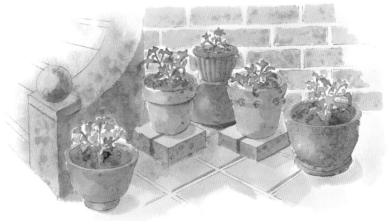

nicotiana knot garden

Knot gardens—contained and given form by clipped box hedges—add timeless style to any outdoor area, whatever its size. The permanent hedge planting can be enlivened by changing the content of the sections of the knot garden, and the easiest way to do this is by using containers. In winter and spring, daffodils or hyacinths will add welcome color, while in the summer bedding plants can be used. Here the tall, fragrant *Nicotiana sylvestris*, known as flowering tobacco, has been used to add another sensory dimension to the planting.

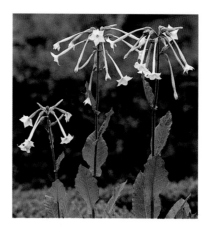

materials & equipment

8 medium pots, about 15 in (38 cm) in diameter
1 large pot, about 20 in (50 cm) in diameter
potting compost
2 buckets of gravel or small stones
plywood for templates
well-rotted organic material

spade
fork
rake
pegs and string
trowel
shears
saw and drill

11 *Nicotiana sylvestris* plants
6 box plants (*Buxus sempervirens* 'Suffruticosa') per 3 ft (1 m) of hedging
well-rotted organic material

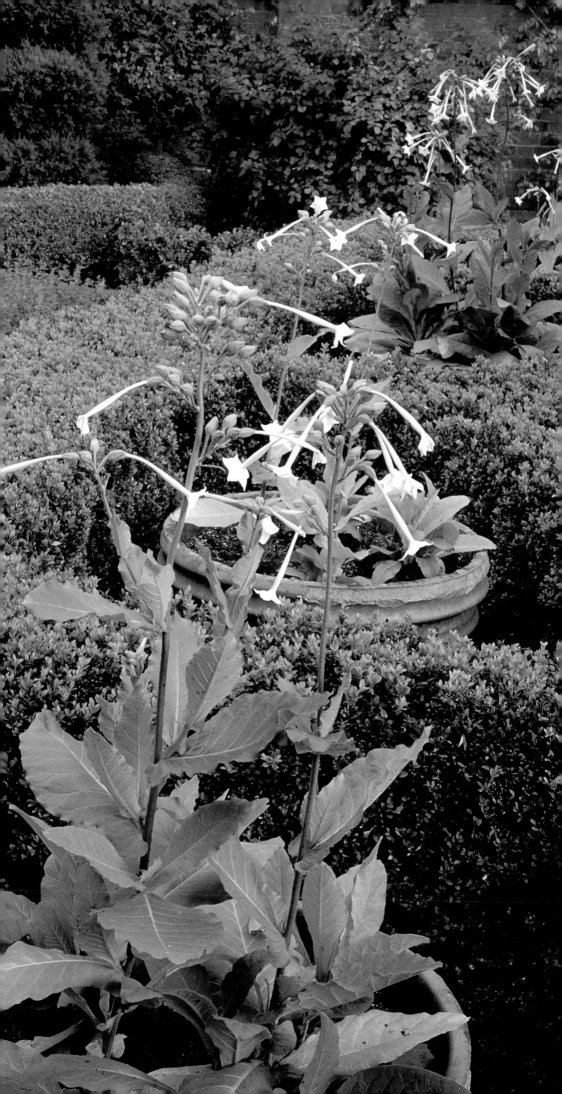

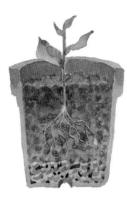

6 planting containers for the nicotiana

To improve drainage, fill the pots with gravel or sharp stones to a depth of 2 in (5 cm). Fill with compost and firm in the nicotiana plant—one in each medium sized pot, and three in the large central pot. Plant the central pot *in situ*—it will be heavy when full.

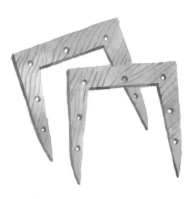

7 shaping the hedge

To give the box hedges a tapered shape, cut two templates out of plywood. The edges of the templates should be pointed so they can be stuck into the ground. Drill holes in each template to form a pattern that matches the intended cross-section of the hedge.

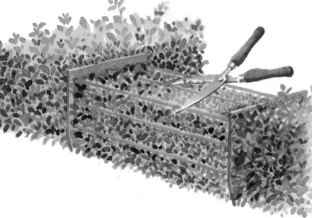

8 trimming the hedge

Place the templates over the hedge; thread strings through the holes and pull them tight. Use the strings as a guide for cutting. Power clippers make for quick work, but hand shears provide more control.

9 care and maintenance

The gaps around the pots can be filled with bedding plants; alternatively, the bare soil can be compacted with a roller and covered with gravel. The containers will need watering every day.

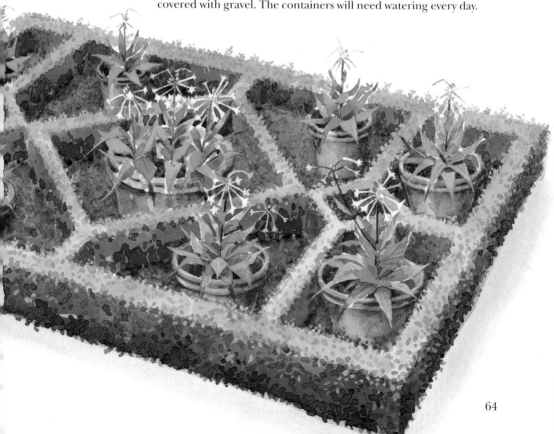

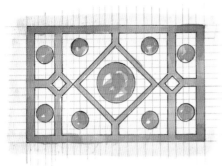

1 planning

Before starting work, carefully draw out the knot garden on graph paper so that your plan can be easily transferred to the ground. The box hedges may take five years or more to reach maturity, so mistakes at this stage are costly. The plot shown here is 8 x 16 ft (2.4 x 4.8 m), but the plan can be modified to suit the space you have available and the shapes you want to create.

2 ground preparation

Dig the plot thoroughly, removing all weeds and incorporating plenty of well-rotted manure. Be sure to prepare the whole plot, not just the run of the hedges, because the planting will be *in situ* for many years.

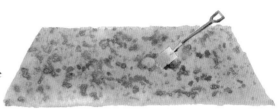

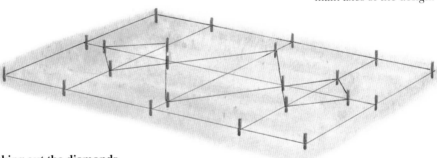

3 marking the main axes

Transfer your drawn plan to the ground with pegs and string. To make sure the pattern is geometric, first mark out the edges of the planting area and the four main axes of the design.

4 marking out the diamonds

Place pegs at suitable intervals along the main strings and then run further lengths of string around these to delineate the diamond shapes of the knot garden. At this stage, check very carefully that the pattern is symmetrical.

5 planting the hedge

Set out the box plants at 6 in (15 cm) intervals along the guide strings. Firm in and water. If the area is exposed to wind, use wind-break netting to reduce its effect until the plants are established.

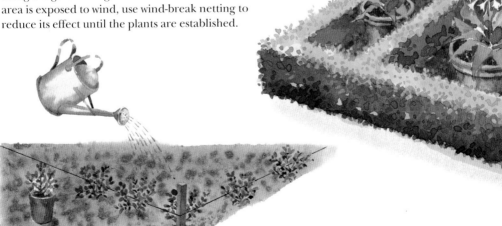

spring window box

Window boxes are a cheerful addition to any house and are
particularly welcome in spring when the fresh colors of early
flowering bulbs cut through the winter gloom. Fill the window box
with a variety of plants—some tall, some trailing, some with patterned
foliage—and be sure to use some scented varieties. The spring
fragrance will waft in through the window, bringing the garden
right into the room.

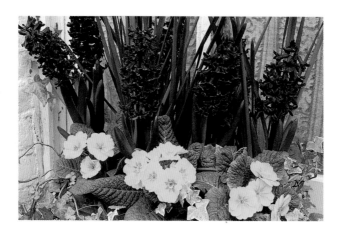

materials & equipment

terra-cotta or wooden window box
broken pots or small pieces of irregular stone
potting soil

trowel
watering can
eye bolts
galvanized wire

Narcissus 'Martinette' x 5
Hyacinthus 'Blue Jacket' x 4
Primula yellow varieties x 3
Hedera helix 'Adam' x 2

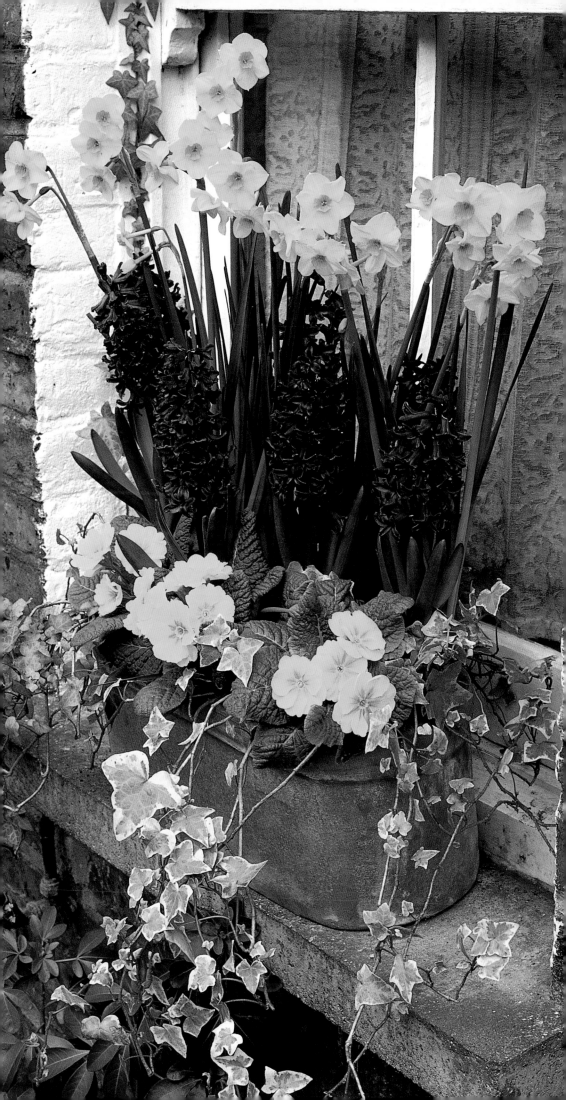

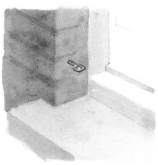

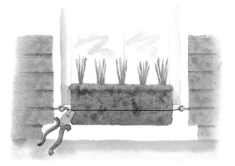

6 safety

The box should be firmly secured to prevent its falling and causing injury. First, screw two eye bolts into either side of the window frame or wall, using a drill and wall plugs if necessary.

7 securing the box

Using a pair of pliers, firmly attach galvanized wire to each eye bolt, stretching it taut around the front of the window box to prevent it from tipping forward.

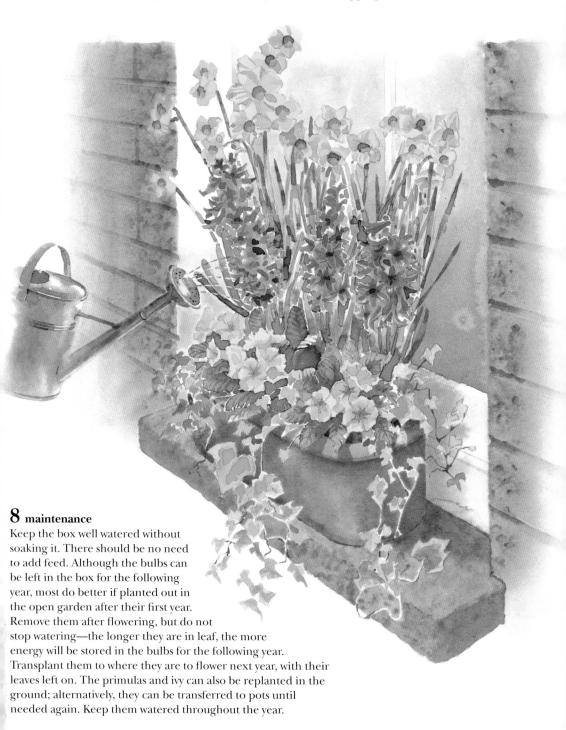

8 maintenance

Keep the box well watered without soaking it. There should be no need to add feed. Although the bulbs can be left in the box for the following year, most do better if planted out in the open garden after their first year. Remove them after flowering, but do not stop watering—the longer they are in leaf, the more energy will be stored in the bulbs for the following year. Transplant them to where they are to flower next year, with their leaves left on. The primulas and ivy can also be replanted in the ground; alternatively, they can be transferred to pots until needed again. Keep them watered throughout the year.

1 choosing the window box

There are many shapes and sizes of box available from nurseries, ranging from the rustic terra-cotta to the ultra-modern plastic or metal. Some plastic boxes have an integral reservoir, which cuts down on watering. Wooden boxes must be coated with preservative before planting.

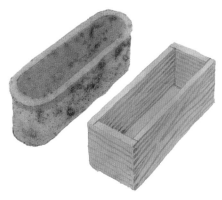

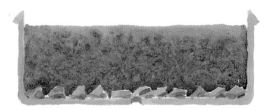

2 filling the box

The window box should be provided with good drainage. Place a layer of broken clay pots, tiles, or small stones in the bottom of the box and fill with a good quality potting soil, which should be firmed down gently but not compacted. To help reduce watering frequency, add water-retaining crystals or granules to the compost. This will absorb large quantities of water, releasing it as the roots require. Follow the instructions on the packet.

3 planting the bulbs

The bulbs are best planted in the autumn when they are dormant—this allows more plants to be fitted in. Plant five narcissus bulbs at the back of the container; their tops should be at a depth of about 4 in (10 cm) below the soil surface. Then plant four hyacinth bulbs so that their tops are just below the surface; they can slightly overlap the narcissus bulbs—there will still be enough room for the leaves and flower shoots of the narcissus to emerge.

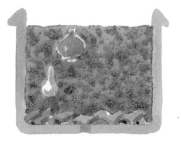

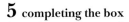

4 planting the primulas and ivy

Plant three primulas in the front of the container, setting them at the same depth as they were in their original pots; then plant two ivies between these and the hyacinths. The primulas can be planted in autumn, but they are not generally available to buy at this time of year; instead, they can be planted in spring just as they are coming into flower. The ivy can be planted at any time.

5 completing the box

Smooth over the top of the soil, adding more if necessary so that the final level is just below the rim of the window box. Fan out the strands of the ivy so that they emerge around and between the primulas. Water well. Cover the compost with a layer of gravel or small stones to make the surface more attractive until it becomes covered in foliage.

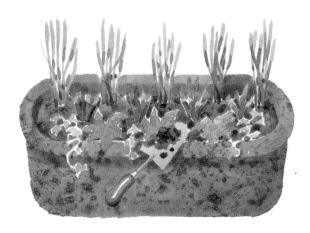

chamomile seat

One of the great joys of creating a garden is the pleasure of sitting and
relaxing surrounded by one's handiwork. This pleasure is even greater
if the garden seat is soft and yielding and produces a wonderful
soothing smell. Chamomile—particularly in its compact, non-flowering
varieties—is the perfect plant to "cover" a seat. It has been used like this
from at least medieval times.

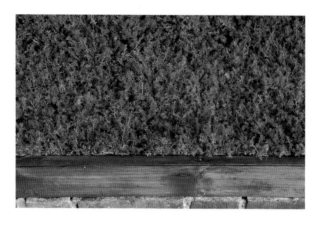

materials & equipment

concrete
approximately 160 bricks
³/₄ in stone
2 wooden planks 1 x 6 in (2.5 x 15 cm), each 6 ft (1.8 m) long
2 wooden planks 1 x 6 in (2.5 x 15 cm), each 2 ft (60 cm) long
galvanized right-angle brackets
galvanized screws
garden soil

pegs and string
measuring tape
spade
shovel
bricklayer's trowel
level
saw
screwdriver
garden trowel
shears

36 chamomile plants (*Chamaemelum nobile* 'Treneague')
6 box plants (*Buxus sempervirens*)
well-rotted organic material

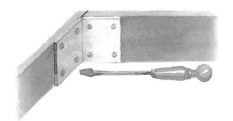

6 making the seat frame

Make a deep wooden frame 2 x 6 ft (60 cm x 1.8 m). This should be made of treated planks 1 x 6 in (2.5 x 15 cm), held together at the corners by galvanized right-angle brackets to give the frame rigidity.

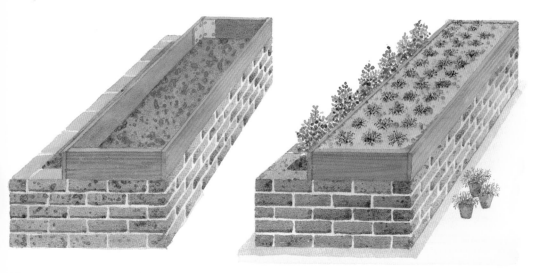

7 filling the frame

Place the frame on top of the bricks. It should be flush to the outside of the brickwork at the ends and front, with a 12 in (30 cm) gap at the back. Fill with earth, topping up when the soil settles. The weight of the earth will keep the frame in place, and the filled frame provides a more comfortable seat than bricks alone.

8 planting

Set out individual chamomile plants at 6 in (15 cm) intervals in each direction. For the "back" of the seat, set out young box plants at 12 in (30 cm) intervals between the back edge of the wooden frame and the back of the brickwork. Before planting, add well-rotted organic material to the strip of soil and dig in.

9 care and maintenance

After a few years, the box will fill out to form a dense back for the rich chamomile-covered seat. Clip the box hedge once or twice a year, and trim the chamomile with hand shears to keep it neat and compact.

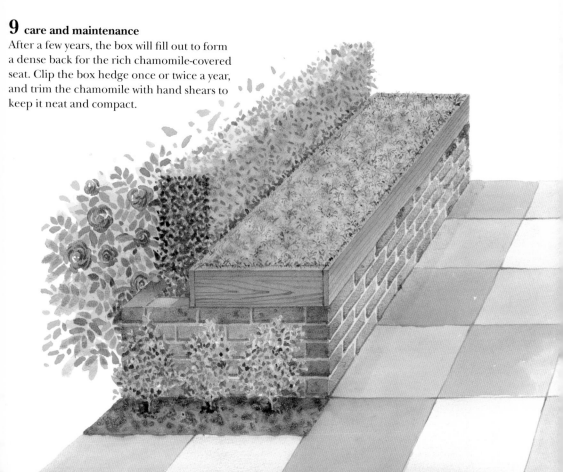

1 marking out the site

On bare ground, mark out the area in which the seat foundations are to be dug. Using pegs and string, make a rectangle 3 x 6 ft (2 x 1.10 m); then mark out a second, smaller, rectangle 10 in (25 cm) within the first.

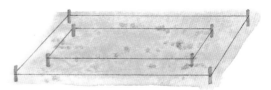

2 digging the foundations

Dig a trench 15 in (40 cm) deep within the guide strings and remove the soil. The foundations and brickwork should ideally be laid in the autumn. This allows time for the soil to be put in place and settle before planting in the spring.

3 building the brick seat

Fill the trench with stone to a depth of 5 in (13 cm) and compact well. Pour and level 4 in (10 cm) of concrete on this base. After seven days, or when the concrete has fully hardened, lay courses of single brickwork on top of the concrete footings, creating a rectangular wall 3 x 6 ft (90 cm x 1.8 m).

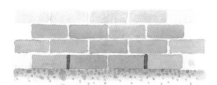

improving drainage
When laying the course of bricks at ground level, omit the vertical pointing between alternate bricks on the front and back walls. This will allow any excess water to drain out from inside.

4 finishing the brick enclosure

The completed brickwork should be approximately five courses high and extend about 15 in (38 cm) above ground level. After seven days, or as soon as the walls have fully set, the brick enclosure should be filled with soil. This job can be left to the spring but is best carried out in autumn to let the winter weather break down the soil.

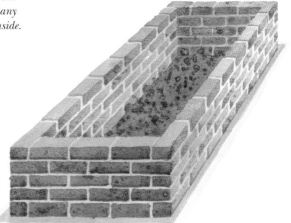

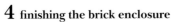

5 filling the enclosure

Pour in a 3 in (8 cm) layer of stone and cover either with permeable horticultural plastic or upturned turf. Fill with earth, firming down as it is filled. Regularly check the soil level during the winter and replenish so that there will be no further settlement once the enclosure is planted in spring.

right A path leading to a secluded arbor is a magical addition to the garden. Sweet peas make an ideal cover for the arbor—they have a long season, which is extended if they are regularly deadheaded.

below Some scented plants are so large that they simply need planting where sufficient space is available. This huge *Philadelphus* hangs over a wall, perfuming the whole length of a path.

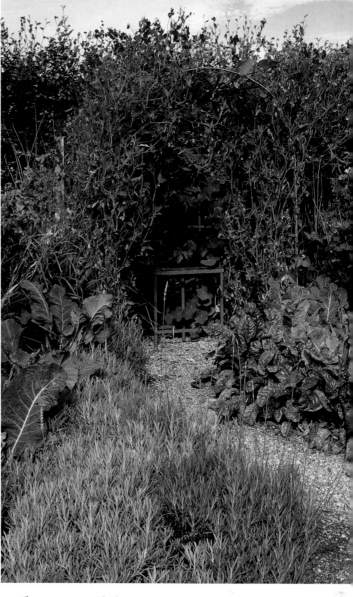

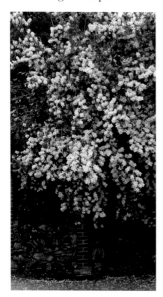

paths and walks
There is something very satisfying about wandering along a path, allowing your fingers to run through rosemary or lavender, releasing fragrance as you pass. For this reason, many scented plants are best placed in beds that fringe walks in the garden. Plants must be chosen with great care; some are freely-scented and best positioned toward the rear of the border; others can be smelled only at close proximity; and others still have foliage that needs to be touched before it releases its scent.

right Paths are excellent places to grow low scented plants. Thyme, for example, is tough enough to be walked on and releases its characteristic scent when trodden underfoot. A crack in the paving is enough to start off a plant, which will soon spread. But beware if walking with bare feet when the thyme is in flower—bees also love the plant!

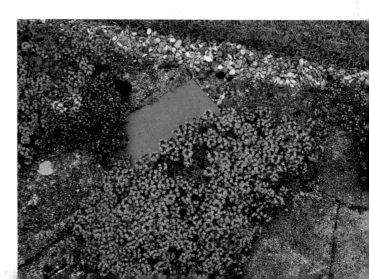

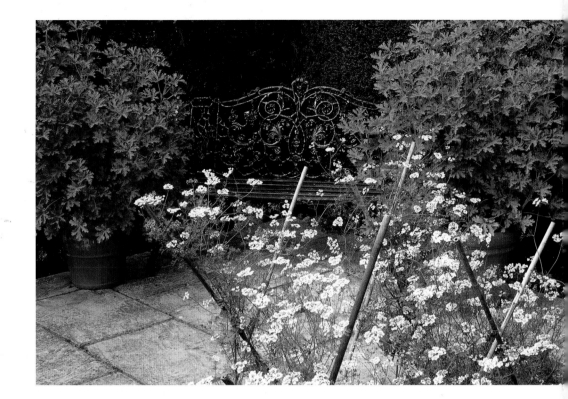

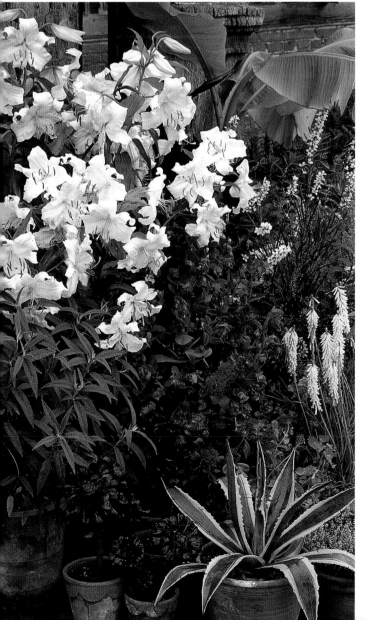

above A shady seat surrounded by scented plants is always difficult to resist. Here lemon-scented pelargoniums and, further away, coriander are planted in pots, which add to the elegance of the setting.

left A wide pathway is an ideal place for setting out a group of pots. Choose a site near a door where the scent will be appreciated by visitors and fill the house through the open door.

below Scented plants are effective singly, but planting a row can create a swathe of fragrance along a path. Take care to choose scents that do not clash, or alternate day and evening scented plants.

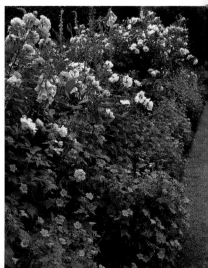

herb path

One of the great joys of walking through a herb garden is being surrounded by a wonderful mixture of scents. On a warm day the air can be full of fragrance. Many herbs release their perfume more strongly when they are slightly bruised, and the action of gently touching them is enough to do this. There can be few things more pleasurable than strolling along a path, brushing herbs as you go, either with your hands or even just the swish of your clothes.

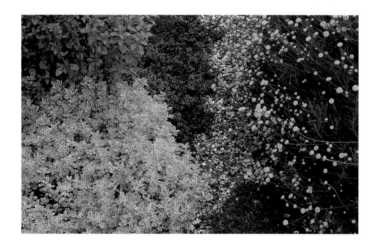

materials & equipment

6–9 house bricks per 3 ft (1 m) of path edging
1 bucket of concrete per 3 ft (1 m) of path edging
gravel for path

spade
tamper
fork
rake
trowel
garden line or pegs and string
brick-laying trowel
mallet
roller

herbs in variety
well-rotted organic material

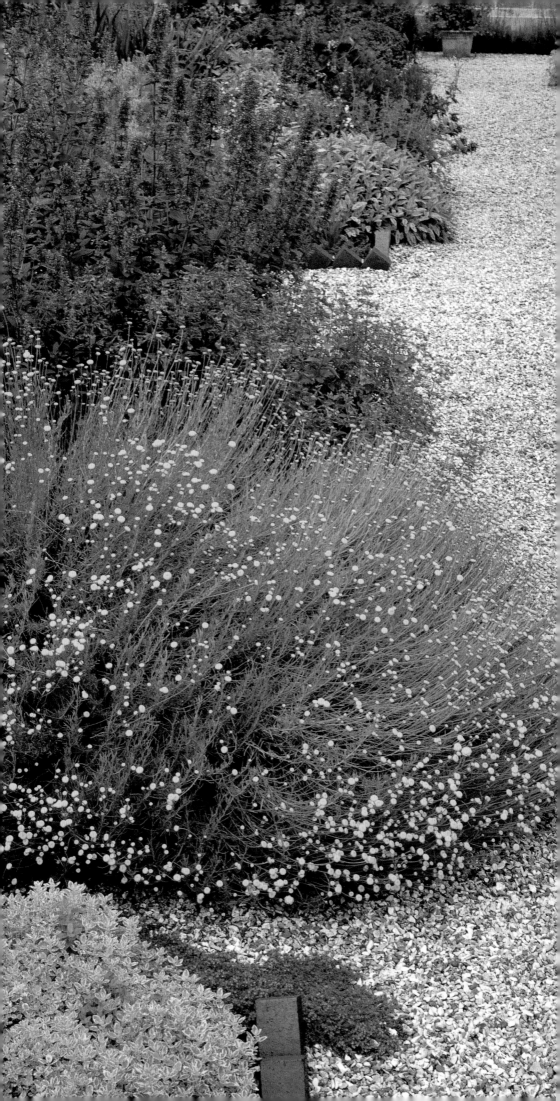

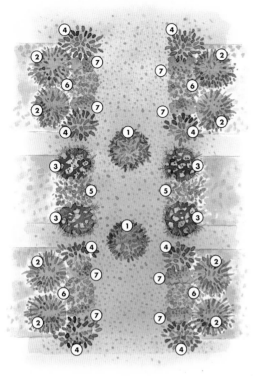

alternative planting

If the paths are laid out in a regular pattern, it can make visual sense to use a more formal planting, perhaps including clipped bay laurel on some of the corners and lemon verbena in pots strategically placed at path junctions. Thyme can be allowed to spread out onto the path so that its fragrance is released when feet accidentally tread on it.

plant list

1 *Aloysia triphylla* x 2 in large pots
2 *Calaminta grandiflora* x 8
3 *Foeniculum vulgare* x 4
4 *Laurus nobilis* x 8
5 *Mentha suaveolens* 'Variegata' x 4
6 *Origanum vulgare* 'Country Cream' x 4
7 *Thymus praecox* 'Coccineus' x 8

5 planting

Prepare the ground, removing all weeds and digging in plenty of well-rotted organic material. Place the plants on the bed, still in their pots, to gain some idea of how the finished arrangement will look. Allow plenty of room for them to spread. Plant the herbs, setting them in the ground to the same depth as they were in their pots. Water thoroughly. If possible, apply a mulch of composted bark, or similar mulch.

plant list

1 *Calaminta grandiflora* x 2
2 *Helichrysum italicum* x 2
3 *Laurus nobile* x 2
4 *Melissa officinalis* x 2
5 *Veronica spicata* 'Heidikind' x 2
6 *Ocimum basilicum* x 2
7 *Origanum vulgare* 'Country Cream' x 2
8 *Petroselinum crispum* x 2
9 *Rosmarinus officinalis* x 2
10 *Salvia officinalis* 'Icterina' x 2
11 *Santolina rosmarinifolia* ssp. *canescens* x 2
12 *Thymus serpyllum praecox*
   'Coccineus' x 2

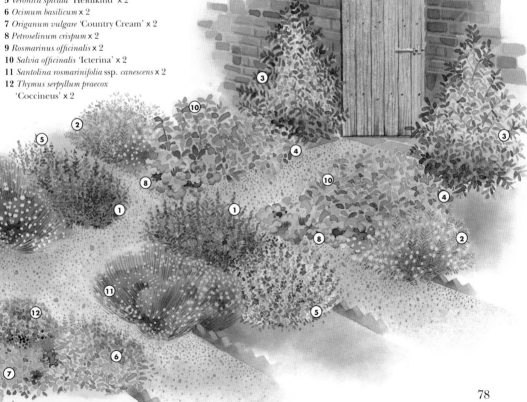

78

1 building the edging
Bricks set diagonally make an attractive and practical edging to a path. The bricks can be set directly into the earth, but for a more permanent edge, dig out a shallow trench, place a layer of concrete in the bottom, and bed in the bricks at your preferred angle.

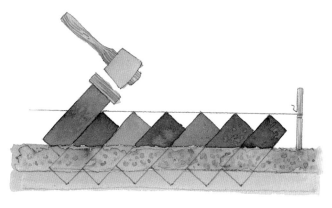

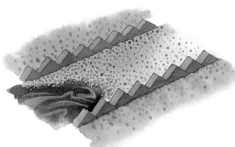

hazel loop edging
Other decorative edgings can be used for the herb path. Low hoops of hazel or similar wood are an informal way of creating a restraining edge. If the herbs are to be kept under tighter control, a higher edging, such as a box hedge, may be appropriate.

2 laying a gravel path
A gravel path is an attractive and relatively cheap form of paving, although it needs to be replenished from time to time. For the simplest path, first lay down the edging and ram down the soil in the path area using a tamper. Pour on gravel to a depth of 1 in (2.5 cm).

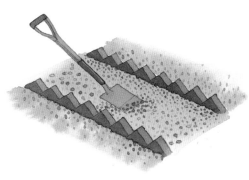

preventing weed growth
Adding a layer of black horticultural polyethylene below the gravel helps prevent weed growth, but the path itself is less solid because its bottom layers cannot be compacted into the earth. However, less gravel is needed when polyethylene is used.

3 rolling
Use a garden roller to compact the loose gravel. Add another 1 in (2.5 cm) layer of gravel and roll in once more. To make a well-bedded path, lubricate the gravel with water when rolling.

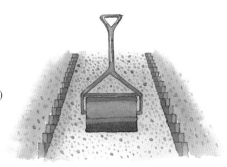

4 raking
Finally add a thin layer of gravel and rake it level. Keep the path weed-free by regularly hoeing or by using a weed killer.

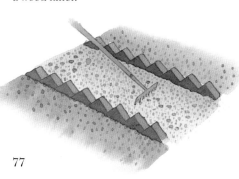

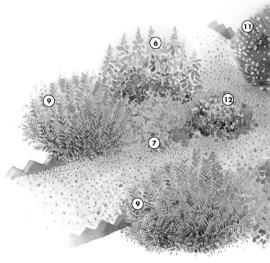

scented chamomile path

There are few experiences that can compare with walking across a spring meadow, engulfed by the fresh scent of the plants around you and beneath your feet. However it is possible, in your own garden, to create a scented environment that is a pleasure to walk through. Chamomile is ideal for this use, because it lends itself to planting in paths and lawns, is fairly resilient underfoot, and releases an unforgettable scent when crushed.

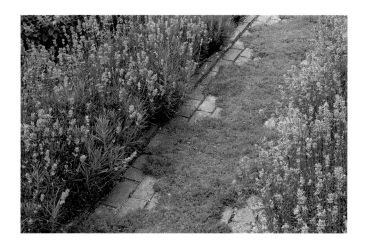

materials & equipment

spade
fork
rake
trowel

25 *Chamaemelum nobile* 'Treneague' plants per square yard (1 m)
well-rotted organic material

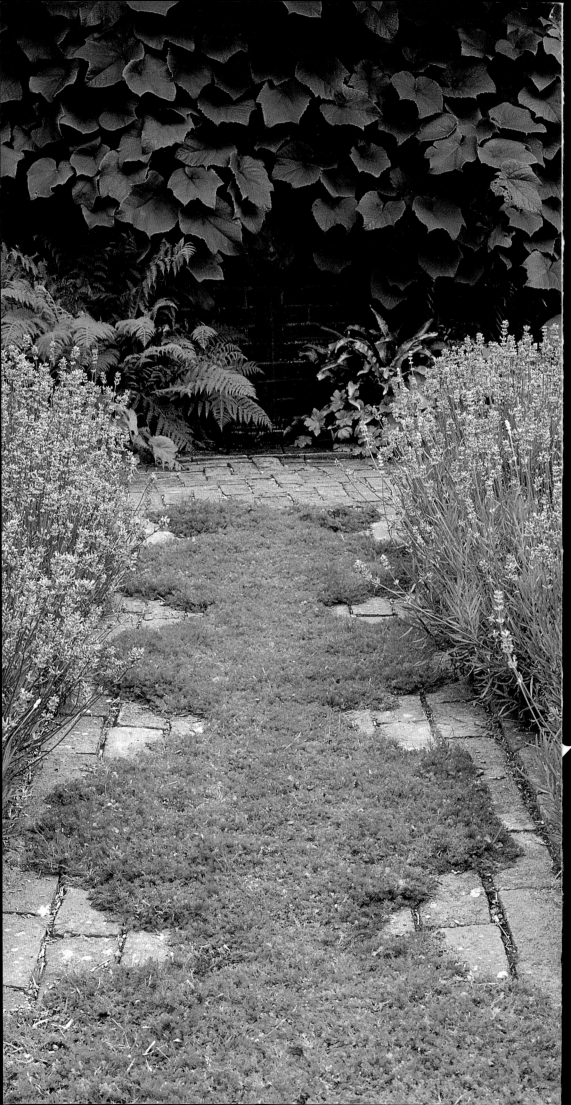

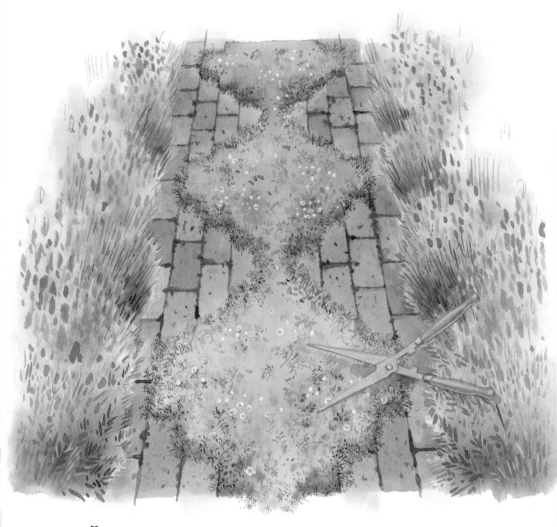

5 maintenance

Chamomile should not need cutting as often as grass, nor should it be cut as tightly, but it responds well to trimming with shears, becoming denser. Larger areas can be cut using a rotary mower on a high setting.

planting for a busy path

Chamomile is not as hard-wearing as grass, and while it will stand the light passage of feet, it should not be used where there is likely to be constant traffic. For busy paths, always leave an alternative paved route.

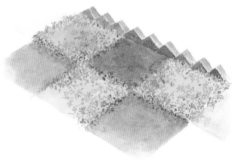

patios and lawns

Chamomile is not usually used for main lawns, but is excellent for small lawns and lightly-used patios. Cobblestones set into the planted area increase its resilience.

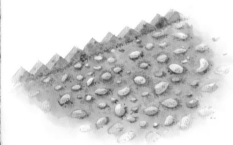

thyme path

Like chamomile, thyme can be planted to break up paved areas, or alternatively in complete carpets. It is very tough and needs just an occasional trim to keep it neat. Don't walk on it with bare feet when it is in flower—there may be bees about!

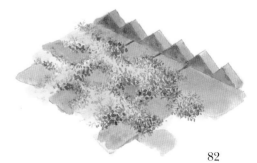

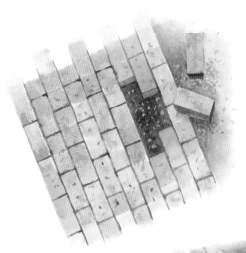

1 the path

Chamomile can be grown into a new path, but it can equally be used to give new life to an old, drab thoroughfare. First lift a few paving stones or bricks from the existing path. These can be taken up at random, but chamomile lends itself to more formal patterns, so it is worth planning out a regular scheme. Chamomile will not take a great deal of hard wear, so if the path is heavily used, leave behind enough bricks on which to walk.

2 preparing the ground

Remove any sand and rubble from beneath the lifted bricks and replace with good loam, working in some organic material, such as well-rotted manure or compost. If the path has been built on a concrete base, this will have to be broken up in the planting areas with a pickaxe before adding fresh soil.

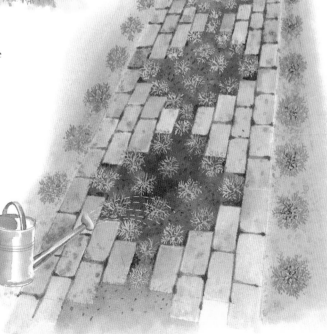

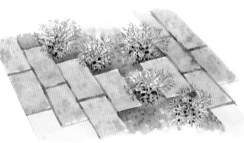

3 planting

In the spring, set out chamomile plants about 9 in (23 cm) apart. It is best to use the low-growing, tufted cultivar *Chamaemelum nobile* 'Treneague' because of its highly-scented foliage and lack of flowers.

4 growing the path

Water the plants thoroughly and avoid walking on them until they have become well established. Keep watered in dry weather and pull up any weeds that germinate in between the plants.

scent-surrounded seat

Gardening should not be all work—you should always allow yourself the time and space to sit down, relax, and enjoy the fruits of your labor. Nothing helps relaxation as much as rich perfumes, and it is a good idea to plant a mixture of fragrant species around seats placed strategically in the garden. Be sure to include plants that flower at different times of year and day so the area is never without perfume.

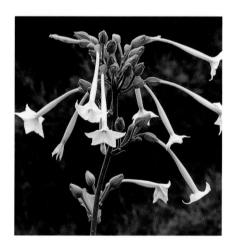

materials & equipment

bench
paving slabs
$3/4$ in stone
cement

spade
fork
tamper
level
garden roller
builder's trowel
garden trowel
rake
pegs and string

plants in variety
well-rotted organic material

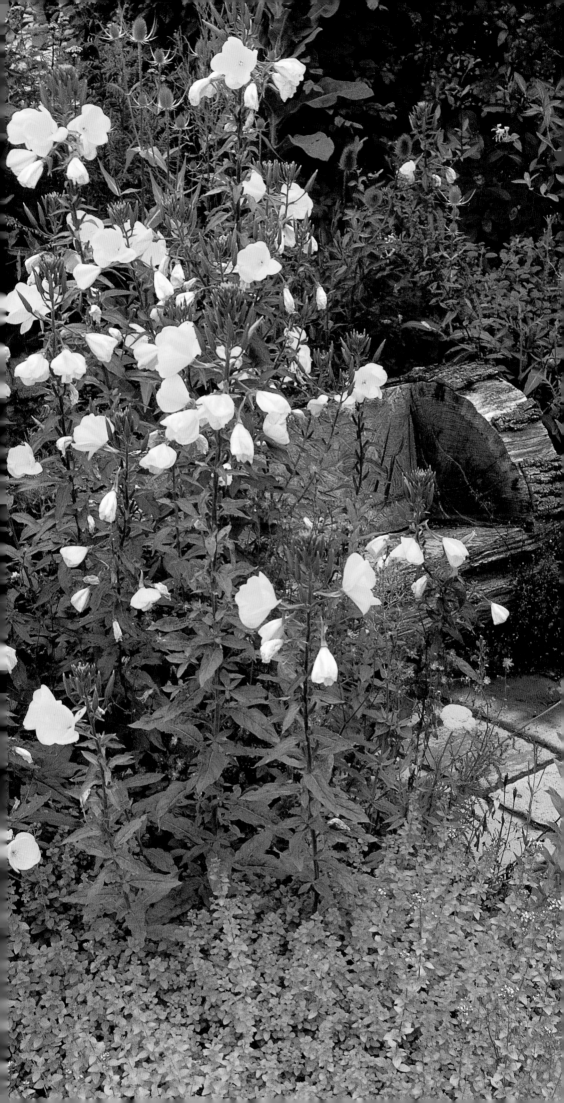

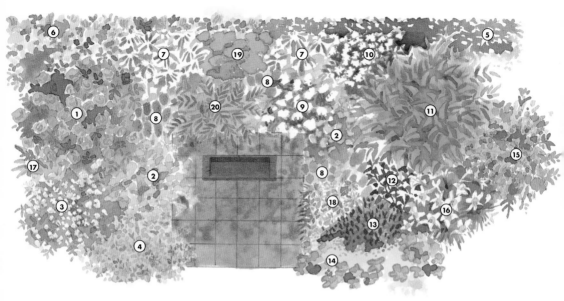

5 arranging the plants

Choose a range of plants that produce scent throughout the year, from daffodils in spring to *Sarcococca* in winter. Mix in some non-scented plants, such as the *Persicaria* and *Dipsacus*, to help balance out the colors and shapes. Shrubs can be underplanted with early-flowering plants.

plant list

1 *Rosa* 'Graham Thomas' × 1
2 *Oenothera biennis* × 3
3 *Philadelphus* 'Manteau d'Hermine' × 1
4 *Origanum vulgare* 'Variegatum' × 1
5 *Jasminum officinale*
6 *Lonicera periclymenum* 'Graham Thomas'
7 *Nicotiana sylvestris* × 3
8 *Dipsacus fullonum* × 3
9 *Phlox paniculata* × 3
10 *Hesperis matronalis albiflora* × 3

11 *Buddleia* × *weyeriana* 'Golden Glow' × 1
12 *Euphorbia dulcis* 'Chameleon' × 1
13 *Persicaria amplexicaulis* × 1
14 *Alchemilla mollis* × 2
15 *Syringa* × *josiflexa* 'Bellicent' × 1
16 *Lillium regale* × 3
17 *Convallaria majalis* × 10
18 *Narcissus* 'Hawera' × 6
19 *Achillea filipendulina*
20 *Sarcococca confusa*

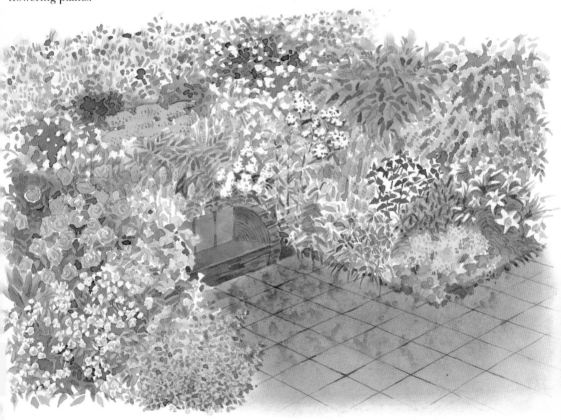

6 care and maintenance

Sweep the paved area regularly and remove any weeds that grow in the cracks. If they become a nuisance over time, apply more cement to the gaps between the slabs. Deadhead the flowers as they fade, and trim the perennials as they die back to increase their vigor.

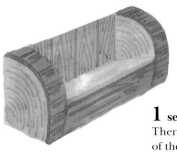

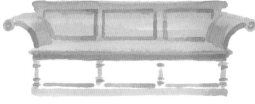

1 selecting the seat

There is a great variety of seat styles available. Consider the location of the seat when choosing—a rustic seat is suitable for cozy garden hideaways, but a more formal and decorative bench works better in open areas, or those that look down a path.

2 paving beneath the seat

Whatever style and size of seat is used, it should sit on a firm base of paving slabs rather than directly on the soil. The paved area should be at least 18 in (45 cm) wider than the bench at the back and sides, and about 4 ft (1.2 m) wider at the front, to give adequate room for a table, or just to stretch your legs. First mark the area to be paved with pegs and string. Dig out the soil to a depth of 6 in (15 cm). Fill with a 4 in (10 cm) layer of stone and ram it down well.

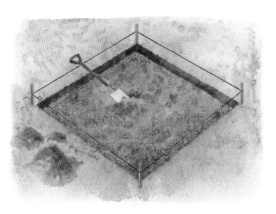

3 laying the paving slabs

On the stone, pour five "blobs" of cement, one in each corner and one in the middle of the resting position of each paving slab. Lay the slabs, tamping them down on the cement. Use a level to check that they are level with their neighbors and perfectly flat. As each slab is laid, put a ¹/₂ in (1 cm) thick piece of wood between it and its neighbors to create even gaps. When the cement is dry, remove the wooden spacer boards and fill the gaps with cement.

4 planting

In autumn, thoroughly prepare the soil surrounding the paving slabs by digging, removing weeds, and adding plenty of well-rotted compost. In spring, place each plant in its container on the bed to get some idea of the visual effect. Dig holes and plant, starting at the back of the bed, firming in and watering as you go. Rake over the surface of the bed to remove footprints.

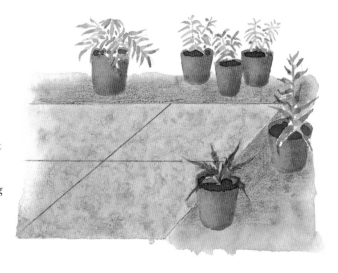

carpet of thyme

Walking across a path dotted with thyme is an experience that is rarely forgotten; at every step the walker is greeted with a waft of the distinctive perfume given off by thyme when its leaves are crushed. Thyme is a very tough plant and will stand being walked upon, making it ideal as a carpeter in the garden. Because it likes well-drained conditions, it can be planted to great effect as drifts on beds of gravel. Such beds are increasingly being used for Mediterranean and aromatic plants, which are becoming popular in dry areas.

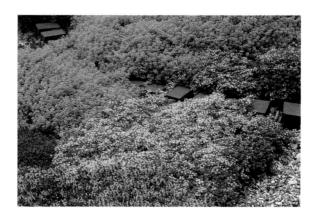

materials & equipment

gravel
treated edging boards, ³/₄ in (2 cm) thick and 4 in (10 cm) wide
decorative stone sets

spade
fork
light garden roller
rake
trowel
pruning shears

thyme in variety:
Thymus serpyllum
T. serpyllum coccineus
T. serpyllum 'Snowdrift'
T. serpyllum 'Minimus'
T. serpyllum 'Pink Chintz'
T. serpyllum 'Doone Valley'
T. pseudolanuginosus
selection of other seedlings

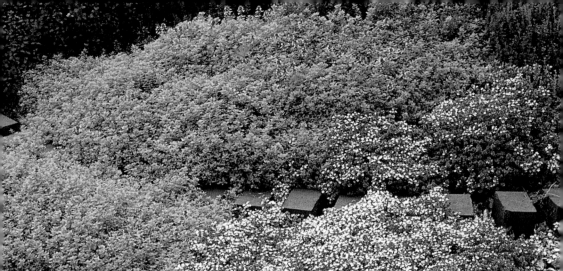

5 thyme varieties

There is a wide range of thymes available that vary in habit, scent, and in the color of their flowers and foliage. Some varieties have golden leaves, while others are green, variegated with yellow, cream, or silver. The flower colors vary from deep purple to white.

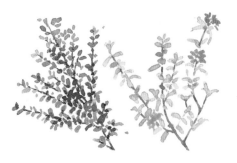

6 planting the thyme

Scrape back the gravel and dig a hole deep enough so that the soil level of the rootball of the thyme is slightly above that of the surrounding soil. Scrape the gravel back around the plants and water well. Plant the thymes about 12 in (30 cm) apart; closer planting will make the carpet form more quickly.

7 care and maintenance

After a few years the thymes may look a bit tired and the center of the plant may die, leaving an ugly bald patch. Dig these plants out in spring and replant any stems that have viable roots. Keep watered until they are established.

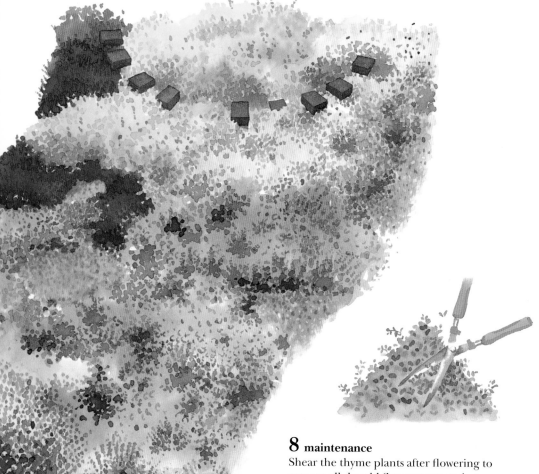

8 maintenance

Shear the thyme plants after flowering to remove all the old flower stems and any straggly growth. In autumn, remove any dead leaves that may have fallen on the thyme to help prevent fungal attack.

1 ground preparation

Dig the plot in the autumn, removing all perennial weeds. Unless the soil is already sandy, incorporate gravel or fine stones to improve the drainage. In spring, rake the bed well.

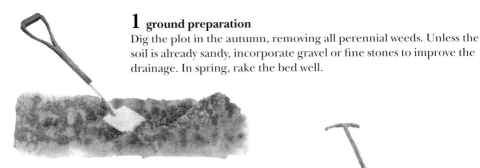

2 flattening and edging the plot

Roll the ground lightly with a garden roller. The depressed area of soil should be edged with treated boards, $^3/_4$ in (2 cm) thick and 4 in (10 cm) wide, before filling with gravel. Sink the boards to a depth at which they are flush with the higher soil level.

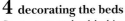

3 gravel beds

Fill the edged bed with a 2 in (5 cm) layer of gravel. Spread the gravel evenly so that it is level with the tops of the edging boards. Wetting the gravel will make it easier to pour. Rake the surface for a neat finish. Natural-colored gravel looks best, but you can also use small stone chippings, which are available in white, pink, or dark gray.

4 decorating the beds

Stone sets embedded in the gravel add visual and textural interest to the beds and can be used to disguise the edging board wherever this is visible. Alternatively, flat stepping stones can be laid in a path through the bed to make access easier.

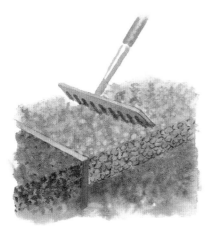

adding texture

If the planting area is not likely to take heavy traffic, then a few boulders, rocks, or even worn pieces of wood can be set into the gravel to give the impression of a dried river bed. To further enhance this effect, the whole area can be sunk down a little by excavating the soil prior to pouring the gravel beds.

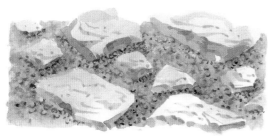

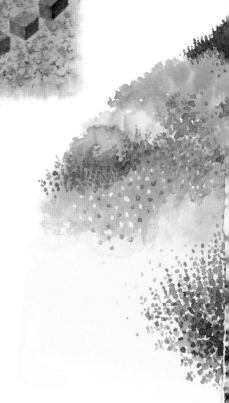

catmint walk

Scented plants are at their most effective when they border a path, spilling over its edges so that they can be crushed underfoot. Anyone strolling along such a path will have the sensation of being enveloped in a tunnel of perfume. This planting works particularly well with a single type of plant, such as catmint or lavender, which gives off a stronger scent when touched; the use of just one perfume further strengthens the sensation of being cocooned in scent for anyone walking down the path.

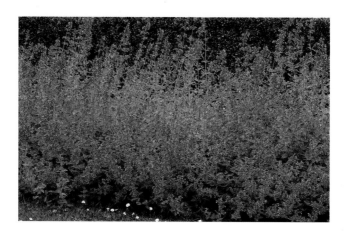

materials & equipment

sharp knife or scalpel
potting soil
spade
fork
rake
trowel
pruning shears
garden line or pegs and string

3 *Nepeta faassenii* plants per yard (1 m)

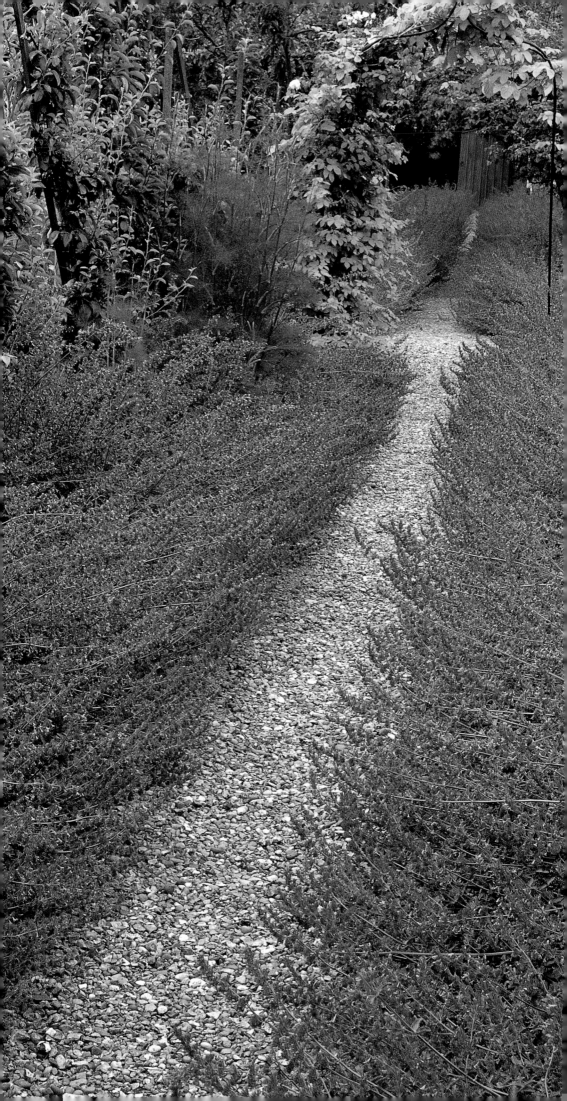

7 preparing the ground

In the autumn, thoroughly prepare the ground, removing any perennial weeds. In spring remove any re-emerging weeds and rake through the soil. Consider the spread of the plants—they should not cover too much of the path or smother plants in the adjacent border, so make sure to place them the right distance apart.

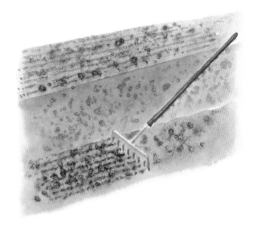

8 planting

Plant parallel to the path using a garden line as a guide. If the path is curved, measure out from the edge of the path each time you plant, using a measuring stick (a piece of wood cut to the right length). Allow about 12 in (30 cm) on either side of each *Nepeta x faassennii* plant; the larger hybrid 'Six Hills Giant' should have no less than 18 in (45 cm) of clearance.

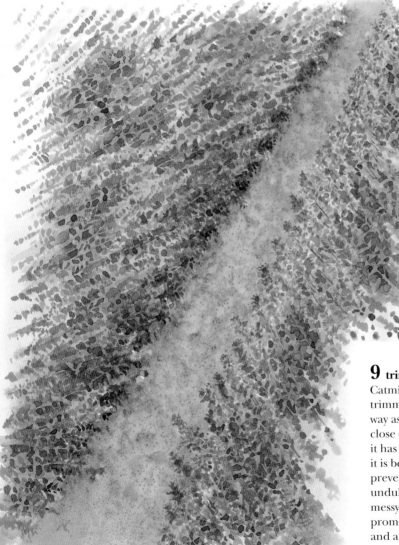

9 trimming

Catmint does not need trimming in the same way as a hedge to keep it close cut. However, after it has finished flowering, it is best to cut it back to prevent it becoming unduly floppy and messy. This cut will promote new growth and a second flowering.

1 acquiring the plants

Lining a path with catmint demands a large number of plants. These are expensive to buy and it is more economical to grow your own from cuttings. Buy a few potted plants in spring and cut them back to promote new growth from the base; this should provide ample cutting material for growing new plants.

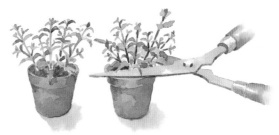

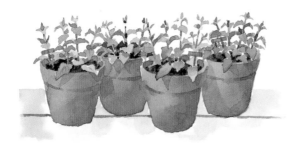

2 taking cuttings

When the new growth reaches a height of 1³/₄ in (4 cm), the shoots can be cut for use as cuttings. Place them in a sealed polyethylene bag and remove them one by one when you are ready to use them.

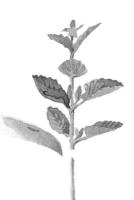

3 cutting the stem

To take a cutting, use a sharp knife or scalpel to slice across the stem just below the lowest leaves. The cutting should be about 1–2 in (2.5–5 cm) in length.

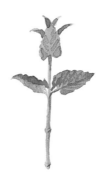

4 removing leaves

Remove the lower leaves of the cutting by slicing them as close as possible to the stem without bruising it. Use either a sharp knife, scalpel, or scissors.

5 potting

Place the cuttings around the edge of a pot filled with potting soil and water well. Place the pot in a propagating tent; alternatively put a polyethylene bag over the pot and plants, making certain that it does not touch the cuttings. Seal the bag around the pot with a rubber band.

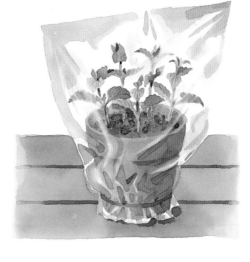

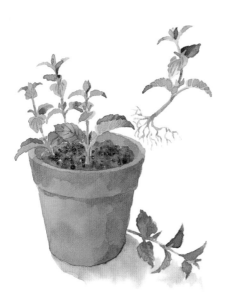

6 removing the cuttings

When the cuttings have rooted (their roots will become visible through the hole in the bottom of the pot), gently remove them and repot individually using a good potting soil. They will be ready to be planted out in the following spring.

plant directory

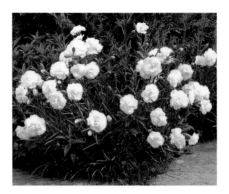

ANNUALS AND BIENNIALS

Annuals can be bought as young plants from nurseries or grown from seed. The latter approach offers a wider choice of plants but is more labor-intensive and time-consuming. Many of the hardy annuals can be sown directly where they are to flower in the spring, and in many cases in the autumn for earlier flowers the next year. They may also be sown in trays.

Most annuals germinate best with a little warmth; a propagating tent is a great help, but the temperature inside most houses is adequate as long as the seedlings get plenty of light, without being exposed to strong direct sunlight. Sow the seeds in a good spotting soil and keep it moist. Once the seed has germinated and the seedlings are large enough to handle, transplant into trays or individual pots. Harden off the plants before planting out. Do not plant out tender plants until after the frosts have passed.

Plant out in well-prepared soil. Keep the plot weeded and well watered. If time allows, deadheading keeps the plants neat and promotes a longer flowering season.

Strictly speaking, some of the following are perennials but are treated in the garden as annuals or biennials.

Calendula officinalis (pot marigold)
Hardy. 18 in (45 cm) high. Yellow to orange flowers appear from spring to autumn. Both flowers and foliage have a very distinctive fragrance. They can be sown where they are to flower in autumn or spring.

Cheiranthus cheiri (English wallflower)
Hardy. 18 in (45 cm) high. The flowers are in a range of colors from yellow and cream to red and purple. They appear in spring and have a very evocative smell. Sow in the open in spring and transplant in autumn.

Heliotropium arborescens (heliotrope)
Half hardy. 18 in (45 cm) high. Deep violet flowers throughout the summer and into autumn have vanilla-like, scent. Sow under glass and transplant after frosts.

Hesperis matronalis (dame's rocket, sweet rocket)
Hardy biennial. 4 ft (1.2 m) high. Flowers are purple or white and emit a wonderful sweet scent, especially at dusk. They appear in early summer. Sow in the open in spring where they are to flower, or in pots and transplant in the autumn. They will self-sow.

Lathyrus odoratus (sweet pea)
Hardy. Up to 6 ft (1.8 m) high. Flowers come in a wide range of colors and varieties. Many, especially the older ones, are highly scented. Good cut flowers. They flower from early summer through to the frosts. Sow in late winter and plant out in early spring or sow in spring for later flowering.

Lobularia maritima (sweet alyssum)
Hardy annual or short-lived perennial. 6 in (15 cm) high. Flowers are mainly white although some are pink to purple. Flowers through summer and into autumn. Sow under glass in spring or a little later outside.

Matthiola bicornis (evening stock)
Half-hardy annual. 12 in (30 cm) high. Lilac flowers with a wonderful, thick, sweet scent in the evenings and after dark. The flowers are not particularly attractive, but worth growing for their scent. Flowers in summer; sow in spring where it is to grow.

Matthiola incana (common stock, Brampton stock)
Hardy biennial or annual. Up to 18 in (45 cm) high. Heavily scented flowers in range of colors. Flowers in late spring to early summer. Sow biennials in summer and over-winter in pots, planting out in spring. Sow annuals in spring in place.

Mirabilis jalapa (four-o'clock)
Half-hardy annual or perennial. Up to 3 ft (90 cm) high. Grown for its lemon-scented flowers, which are trumpet-shaped and come in various shades of pink, yellow, and white. Flowers do not open until late afternoon. Raise from seed sown under glass in spring.

Nicotiana (tobacco plant)
Half-hardy annual. Up to 7 ft (2.1 m) high. A number of different species and cultivars, many of which have a heady evening scent. The scented varieties are mainly white. Sow in spring under glass and plant out after the frosts have passed.

Oenothera biennis (evening primrose)
Hardy biennial. 3 ft (90 cm) high. Yellow flowers have a sweet, slightly astringent smell in the evening. They flower throughout the summer. Sow in spring or summer where they are to flower. They will self-sow.

Pelargonium (geranium—scented leaved varieties)
Tender perennial. Up to 30 in (75 cm) high. Leaves are scented, but (mainly) pink or white flowers are not. Have a long flowering period from early summer until the frosts. Propagate from cuttings.

Petunia
Half-hardy annual. 10 in (25 cm) high, but there are also trailing varieties. Trumpet-shaped flowers are available in a large range of colors that appear over a long period from summer to the end of autumn. The flowers of some varieties are sweetly scented, particularly in the evenings. Sow in spring under glass and plant out once the frosts have passed.

Reseda odorata (mignonette)
Hardy annual. 12 in (30 cm) high. An old-fashioned plant with spikes of small, greenish-yellow flowers, tinged with red, that are often highly scented. If sown successionally, will flower throughout the summer. Sow outside from spring onward.

Viola x *wittrockiana* (pansy)
Hardy annual or short-lived perennial. Up to 10 in (25 cm) high. Many varieties are fragrant. They are available in a wide range of colors and flower in all seasons of the year, depending on zone. Sow under glass.

PERENNIALS

Perennials are available from nurseries but can also be grown from seed or propagated from cuttings or by division. Most have a fragrance of some sort, even if it is only a leafy smell when the foliage is crushed, but some—listed below—are known for their perfume.

Buying from a nursery or propagating from existing plants enable you to check that the plant is a perfumed variety before planting—growing from seed is less certain. Prepare the ground for perennials in the autumn; break down the soil again in spring and remove all weeds just before planting. Avoid planting too tightly because many perennials spread to form clumps. If possible, mulch the ground after planting.

Keep the plot weeded and well watered. Taller plants may need staking, especially if the bed is exposed. Deadheading keeps the plants neat and also prolongs the flowering season. Some plants benefit from being cut to the ground after flowering. At the end of the season, cut down all dying vegetation, weed through the beds, and top-dress with garden compost or farmyard manure.

Agastache foeniculum (hyssop)
3 ft (90 cm) high. A short-lived perennial with anise-scented foliage. Flowers can be mauve, red, pink, or white and appear throughout the summer. Sow in pots in spring and transplant the following spring.

Aponogeton distachyus (water hawthorn)
6 in (15 cm) high. A floating water plant with white flowers that appear throughout the summer and into the autumn. The flowers have a vanilla-like scent in the evening. Propagate by division.

Asphodeline lutea (King's spear)
3 ft (90 cm) high. Flowers are golden stars opening in a spike above narrow gray-green leaves. They flower in early summer and like a hot, sunny position. Propagate by division or from seed.

Calamintha grandiflora (calamint)
12 in (30 cm) high. A low, bushy plant with fragrant foliage and pink flowers in summer. Propagate by division or from seed.

Cestrum parqui
7 ft (2.1 m) high. A shrub-like perennial with yellow flowers. Its summer and autumn flowers have a savory smell during the day and a sweet scent during the evening and night. Slightly tender; can be cut to the ground by frosts, but will regenerate. Propagate by division or cuttings.

Clematis heracleifolia
2 ft (60 cm) high. An herbaceous clematis with small, blue flowers and a strong, sweet scent in the late summer and autumn. Propagate by division and cuttings.

Clematis recta
4 ft (1.2 m) high. An herbaceous clematis with small, strongly-scented, creamy flowers that appear in summer. The purple-leaved form 'Purpurea' is best. Needs support.

Convallaria majalis (lily-of-the-valley)
9 in (23 cm) high. Spikes of fragrant, white bells appear in late spring. Spreads to form a dense carpet. Grows in light shade. Propagate by division.

Cosmos atrosanguineus (chocolate plant)
2 ft (60 cm) high. Dark red flowers that smell of chocolate in warm weather. They appear in late summer. Propagate by division or basal cuttings.

Crambe cordifolia (crambe)
6 ft (1.8 m) high. This plant produces a haze of white, honey-scented flowers in early summer. It is prone to slug attack. Propagate from root cuttings.

Dianthus (pink)
12 in (30 cm) high. Old-fashioned varieties, in particular, are often highly scented, smelling of cloves. They come in a range of whites, pinks, and reds. Old varieties flower in early summer; modern ones throughout summer and autumn. Propagate by cuttings.

Filipendula ulmaria (Queen of the Meadow)
2 ft (60 cm) high. The plumes of creamy-white flowers produced in summer are highly scented. It prefers damp soil. Propagate by division.

Galium odoratum (sweet woodruff)
6 in (15 cm) high. A carpeting woodland plant that smells of new-mown hay. It has white, starry flowers in late spring. Prefers shade. Propagate by division.

Geranium macrorrhizum (bigroot cranesbill)
12 in (30 cm) high. A good carpeting plant that forms a dense ground cover, even in dry shade. The foliage has a strong, sweetish scent when brushed against. The flowers are in various shades of pink and white, and appear in late spring. Propagate by division.

Hemerocallis (daylily)
3 ft (90 cm) high. A number of day lilies have fragrant, trumpet-shaped flowers, mainly in varying shades of yellow, orange, and mahogany, which appear in summer. Will grow in light shade. Propagate by division.

Hosta 'Honeybells' (plantain lily)
2 ft (60 cm) high. Hostas are mainly grown for their foliage, but they also have very attractive, lily-like flowers in either white or blue. This variety has lilac flowers that are distinctly scented. It will grow in shade as well as sun. Propagate by division.

Iris
Up to 3 ft (90 cm) high. Many have fragrant flowers, including *I. unguicularis*, the winter iris. A wide range of colors is available, especially among the bearded irises, which flower in early summer. Most fragrant forms like a sunny position. Propagate by division.

Lunaria rediviva (honesty)
24 in (60 cm) high. A fragrant, perennial form of the annual honesty. It has white flowers tinged with lilac that appear in late spring and early summer. Will grow in sun or light shade. Propagate from seed or division.

Lupinus polyphyllus (lupine)
Up to 4 ft (1.2 m) high. The old-fashioned flowers form distinctive spikes and have an alluring, peppery smell. Flowers are in all shades; they appear in early summer and again later if the old spikes are cut off just after flowering. They thrive in full sun and are best grown from seed but can be divided.

Nepeta (catmint)
Up to 3 ft (90 cm) high. Grown for the wonderful haze of flowers produced, as well as for the fragrant foliage. Flowers are lavender blue and are produced in long, arching spikes in summer and again in autumn if cut back after flowering. Grown from seed sown in spring, basal cuttings taken in spring, or careful division at the same time of year.

Oenothera (evening primrose)
Up to 5 ft (1.5 m) high. Short-lived perennials with mainly yellow, but also white or pink flowers that have a distinctive fragrance, which intensifies into the evening. They appear during the summer and often well into the autumn. Grow in the sun. Propagate from seed.

Paeonia (peony)
Up to 3 ft (90 cm) high. There are a large number of peonies available, many with fragrant flowers, principally white or pink. They have a relatively short flowering season that extends from late spring to early summer. The cultivars can be propagated by division, while species can also be increased from seed.

Petasites (butterbur)
Flowers up to 10 in (25 cm) high; leaves up to 3 ft (90 cm). These winter-flowering plants have intensely sweet scented flowers. The flowers appear before the leaves, which in some species can become very long and smother all below. They are rampant spreaders and are not for the small garden. Increase by division.

Phlox
Up to 4 ft (1.2 m) high. The flowers of forms of the border phloxes *P. maculata* and *P. paniculata* have a distinctive and attractive sweet peppery smell, especially when the weather is warm. The flowers appear during the summer months. They are normally grown in the sun but will tolerate a little light shade. Propagate by division or root cuttings.

Polygonatum (Solomon's seal)
3 ft (90 cm) high. The arching stems carry small, tubular flowers in spring that emit a slight scent, most noticeable in warm conditions. This fresh-looking plant grows most successfully in shady conditions. Increase by division.

Primula (primrose)
Up to 2 ft (60 cm) high. A large genus of plants of which many are scented. Most typical of the group are the English primrose (*P. vulgaris*) and the cowslip (*P. veris*). Both produce their yellow flowers in spring. There are also many colored hybrids, especially of the polyanthus group. In the early summer, the taller Himalayan cowslip (*P. sikkimensis*) produces scented yellow flowers. Most primulas do best in light shade and moist soil. Increase by division or seed.

Romneya coulteri (California tree poppy)
6 ft (2 m) high. A shrubby perennial with huge, fragrant, pure white flowers with a bright golden central boss in summer. Like most poppies, the petals are like crumpled tissue paper. Beautiful as they are, they can be rampant and so are not suitable for the small garden unless contained. Cut back old stems in spring. Plant in the sun. Propagate from root cuttings.

Smilacina racemosa (false Solomon's seal)
3 ft (90 cm) high. A relative of the Solomon's seal with clusters of creamy white, lemon-scented, frothy flowers in spring. Prefers a lightly shaded site. Propagate by division.

Tellima grandiflora (fringe cups)
2 ft (60 cm) high. Grown mainly for its decorative qualities but the flowers are also fragrant. They are small whitish-green cups, fringed with red and held in tall airy spikes. They appear from late spring into early summer. It is a good plant for light shade, although it will grow in sun if the soil is reasonably moist. Propagate from seed.

Verbena bonariensis
Up to 5 ft (1.5 m) high. Tall, wiry plant with flat heads of purple, slightly fragrant flowers, much loved by butterflies. They appear in late summer and autumn. There is a shorter 12 in (30 cm) high version in *V. corymbosa*, which has bluer flowers and a tendency to spread. Propagate from seed.

Viola odorata (sweet violet)
6 in (15 cm) high. Typically these plants have violet-blue flowers with a distinctive scent. They are also available in other shades of blue as well as white, purple, and purplish-pink. They will grow in sun if the soil is reasonably moist, but do best in light shade and cooler climates. Increase by division or from seed.

Yucca

Up to 8 ft (2.5 m) high. These are shrubby perennials with narrow leaves and tall spikes covered in fountains of creamy-white bells. The flowers are sweetly fragrant and appear in summer through to the autumn. The leaves can be stiffly pointed and very sharp. Grow in full sun. Propagate by division or root cuttings.

HERBS

Most herbs are readily available from nurseries, although they are often inadequately labeled and may simply be called "mint" (for example) with no variety specified. Crush a leaf to see if you like the smell and taste before buying. Most varieties of herbs need to be propagated vegetatively, but species can be grown from seed; the latter are generally available from seed merchants and horticultural outlets.

Herbs may be in position for several years so it is imperative that the ground is well-prepared. Dig in as much organic material as possible and remove all weeds; if these are not totally cleared, the whole herb garden may later have to be removed, cleaned of weeds, and replanted. The best time to dig is in the autumn—the weather will break down the soil and the remains of weeds before planting begins in the spring.

Plant at the same depth as the herbs were in their containers. Rake over the surface and water in. Cut back flowering stems before they set seed unless you want to collect the seed for culinary or propagation purposes. On perennial plants, cut back the foliage stems as the leaves begin to look tired so that new, fresh foliage is produced. Cut off all dead stems in autumn or spring, before new growth starts.

Seed can be sown in spring under glass or in the open soil. Tender herbs should not be planted out until the frosts have passed. Many perennials can be either divided or increased from basal cuttings in spring, and shrubby ones from cuttings in summer.

Allium schoenoprasum (chive)

Perennial bulb. 12 in (30 cm) high. Grown for their leaves. Buy container plants or divide existing ones in spring. Plant out 8 in (20 cm) apart. Harvest as required. The leaves can be dried or frozen for storage. Attractive pink-purple flowers in early summer. Good plant for edging.

Aloysia triphylla (lemon verbena)

Perennial. Up to 4 ft (1.2 m) high, or taller in warm climates. Grown for its strongly lemon-scented leaves. Harvest fresh leaves at any time. Dry leaves for storage. Good plant for growing in containers.

Anethum graveolens (dill)

Annual. Up to 5 ft (1.5 m) high. Grown for its leaves and seed. Sow where it is to grow from spring onward. Thin to 10 in (25 cm) intervals. Harvest leaves when young and tender, and seed when ripe. Dry leaves and seeds for storage.

Angelica archangelica (angelica)

Biennial or short-lived perennial. 3–8 ft (1–2.5 m) high. Grown for stem, seed, and leaves. Sow in autumn or spring in a pot or where it is to grow. Plant or thin to 3 ft (90 cm) intervals. Harvest stems in summer, seed in late summer/autumn, and leaves before flowering. The leaves can be dried for storage and the stems candied. An attractive architectural plant.

Anthriscus cerefolium (chervil)

Annual. 15 in (38 cm) high. Grown for its leaves, which resemble those of parsley. Sow where it is to grow from spring onward for a continuous supply. Thin to 8 in (20 cm). Harvest before flowering.

Artemisia dracunculus (tarragon)

Tender/hardy perennial. 2 ft (60 cm) high. Grown for its leaves, which have a minty-anise flavor. Buy container plants or take cuttings from an existing plant in summer. Plant at 18 in (45 cm) intervals. Harvest leaves as required. The leaves can be dried or frozen for storage.

Borago officinalis (borage)

Annual. 30 in (75 cm) high. Grown for its flowers and young leaves. Sow seeds in a pot or where it is to grow. Thin to or plant out at 12 in (30 cm) intervals. Harvest leaves young and flowers when required. Flowers can be frozen in ice cubes or crystallized. Very attractive blue flowers.

Calendula officinalis (pot marigold)

Hardy annual. Grown for its flowers (which can be used as a substitute for saffron) and leaves. Sow where it is to grow in autumn or spring. Thin to 12 in (30 cm) intervals. Harvest as required. Flowers can be dried for storage. Bright addition to a herb garden.

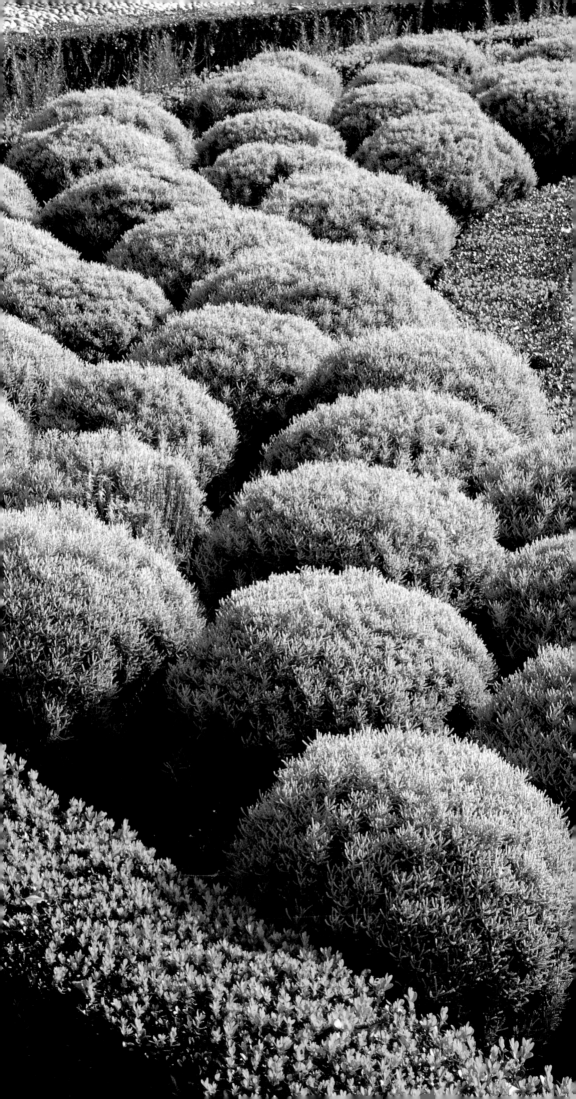

Carum carvi (caraway)
Annual or biennial. 2 ft (60 cm) high. Grown
for its seed and leaves. Thin seedlings in
spring to 8 in (20 cm) apart. Harvest leaves
when young and seed in late summer when
ripe. The seeds can be dried for storage.

Chamaemelum nobile (chamomile)
Hardy perennial. 10 in (25 cm) high.
Grown for its leaves. Sow in spring in pots,
or divide existing plants in spring and plant
out at 6 in (15 cm) intervals. Harvest leaves
at any time. The leaves can be dried for
storage. The variety 'Treneague' is good
for lawns.

Coriandrum sativum (coriander)
Biennial. 2 ft (60 cm) high. Grown for its
leaves and seeds. Sow in autumn or spring
where it is to grow and thin to 8 in (20 cm)
intervals. Harvest leaves as required and
seeds when ripe. Dry seeds and freeze leaves
for storage.

Foeniculum vulgare (fennel)
Hardy perennial. 7 ft (2 m) high. Grown for
its leaves and seed. Sow in spring in pots or
where it is to grow. Thin or plant out to
2 ft (60 cm) intervals. Harvest leaves as
required and seed when ripe. Dry seeds and
freeze leaves for storage. Attractive foliage,
especially in its bronze form 'Purpureum.'
Avoid letting it go to seed or it will self-sow.

Hyssopus officinalis (hyssop)
Hardy shrub. 2 ft (60 cm) high. Grown for
its leaves. Buy as a container plant or take
cuttings from an existing plant in summer.
Plant at 2 ft (60 cm) intervals. Harvest leaves
as required. The leaves can be dried for
storage. Attractive foliage and violet or white
flowers. Suitable for hedges in herb gardens
or knot gardens.

Laurus nobilis (bay)
Hardy evergreen shrub. Up to 15 ft (4.5 m)
high. Grown for its leaves. Buy as a container
plant or take cuttings in late summer and
plant out resulting plants when big enough.
Can be topiaried. Harvest leaves as required.
Dried leaves are sweeter than fresh ones.

Levisticum officinale (lovage)
Hardy perennial. 7 ft (2 m) high. Grown for
its leaves and seed. Buy a plant or sow seed in
autumn. Plant out at 30 in (75 cm) intervals.
Harvest leaves as needed and seed when ripe.
Dry or freeze leaves for storage.

Melissa officinalis (lemon balm)
Hardy perennial. 3 ft (90 cm) high. Grown
for its leaves. Buy a container plant or divide
an existing plant in spring. Plant out at
2 ft (60 cm) intervals. Harvest leaves as
required. The leaves can be dried for
storage. Cut back before it seeds or it could
spread and become a nuisance.

Mentha (mint)
Hardy perennial. 2 ft (60 cm) high. The
different varieties of mint are grown for their
leaves; variegated varieties make attractive
border plants, but must be surrounded by
vigorous neighbors. Buy a container plant
or divide an existing plant. Plant at 12 in
(30 cm) intervals. Rampant spreaders so
best contained below soil level. Harvest
leaves as required. The leaves can be dried
or frozen for storage. There is a wide
variety of forms available; some are
more decorative than others, but all have
scented foliage.

Monarda didyma (bergamot)
Hardy perennial. 3 ft (90 cm) high. Grown
for its leaves. Buy as container plant or divide
an existing plant in spring. Plant at 2 ft (60
cm) intervals. Harvest leaves as required.
The leaves can be dried for storage. Very
attractive red, pink, white, or purple flowers.

Myrrhis odorata (sweet cicely)
Hardy perennial. 30 in (75 cm) high. Grown
for its seeds and leaves. Sow in autumn or
spring either in pots or where it is to grow.
Plant out at or thin to 2 ft (60 cm) intervals.
Harvest leaves while they are young and seed
either while still green or when fully ripe.
Dry unripe seed for storage. Attractive
hedgerow plant.

Ocimum basilicum (basil)
Tender annual. 8 in (45 cm) high. Grown for
its leaves. Sow under glass or after frosts
where it is to grow. Plant at or thin to 8 in (20
cm) intervals. Harvest leaves as required.
The leaves can be dried for storage. Varieties
available include purple-leaved forms.

Origanum (marjoram, oregano)
Annual or perennial. 2 ft (60 cm) high.
Grown for its leaves. Grow from seed in
spring or by division of existing plants. Plant
out at 18 in (45 cm) intervals. Harvest as
required. The leaves can be dried or frozen
for storage. The golden form *O. vulgare*
'Aureum' is particularly attractive.

Petroselinum crispum (parsley)
Biennial. 12 in (30 cm) high. Grown for its
leaves. Sow in spring where it is to grow or in
pots. Thin or plant out at 9 in (23 cm)
intervals. Harvest leaves as required. The
leaves can be dried or frozen for storage.
The curled-leaved forms make very
decorative edging.

Pimpinella anisum (anise)
Annual. 12–16 in (30–45 cm) high. Grown
for its seed and leaves. Sow where it is to
grow in spring. Thin to 8 in (20 cm). Harvest
as required. Seeds can be dried and stored.

Rosmarinus officinalis (rosemary)
Hardy evergreen shrub. Up to 6 ft (1.8 m)
high. Grown for its leaves. Buy a container
plant or take cuttings in summer. Plant out
in spring at 5 ft (1.5 m) intervals. Harvest
leaves as required. The leaves can be dried
for storage. Plant where the leaves can be
easily touched so that their scent is released.
Has attractive blue flowers in spring.

Salvia officinalis (sage)
Hardy evergreen shrub. 2 1/2 ft (75 cm) high.
Grown for its leaves. Buy a container plant or
take cuttings in summer. Plant out in spring
at 3 ft (90 cm) intervals. Harvest leaves as
required. The leaves can be dried for
storage. Plant near a path where its fragrant
foliage can be appreciated.

Satureja hortensis (summer savory)
Annual. 18 in (45 cm) high. Grown for its
leaves. Sow in spring in pots or where it is to
grow. Plant at out or thin to 9 in (23 cm)
intervals. Harvest leaves as required. The
leaves can be dried for storage.

Satureja montana (winter savory)
Hardy shrub. 18 in (45 cm) high. Grown for
its leaves. Buy as a container plant or take
cuttings from an existing plant in summer.
Plant out at 18 in (45 cm) intervals. Harvest
leaves as required. The leaves can be dried
for storage.

Thymus vulgaris (thyme)
Hardy shrub. Up to 12 in (30 cm) high.
Grown for its leaves. Buy as a container plant
or take cuttings from an existing plant in
summer. Plant out at 12 in (30 cm) intervals.
Harvest leaves as required. The leaves can be
dried for storage. A tough plant suitable for
planting between paving slabs, in rock
gardens, on walls, and in containers.

BULBS

Bulbs are often overlooked when planning
scented plantings, but many have a
wonderful perfume, especially in warm
weather. Bulbs are particularly useful in small
gardens because they take up little space and
most have a short season during which they
show above ground, which means that they
can be used to plant under or between other
plants. Many bulbs have unattractive leaves,
especially when they begin to wither, but this
can be disguised by planting them among
other plants. They are also useful for
providing color and fragrance in the spring
while other plants are still thinking about
waking up.

Bulbs need to be planted while they are
dormant; in most cases, this means autumn,
although autumn-flowering bulbs should be
planted in spring. The rule of thumb for
planting is to set the bulb in to a depth below
the soil equal to twice the height of the bulb
itself. Mark their position carefully because
bulbs are invisible once the foliage dies down
and are easily destroyed by accident.

Amaryllis belladonna (Belladonna lily)
18 in (45 cm) high. An autumn-flowering
bulb, the flowers of which appear well before
the leaves. The flowers are bright rose-pink
flared trumpets with a white center. They like
a warm position.

Cardiocrinum giganteum (Himalayan lily)
Up to 8 ft (2.5 m) high. This is one of the
tallest of bulbs, with a large spike of white
trumpet flowers in mid-summer. The bulbs
take several years to reach flowering size,
and, unfortunately, die after flowering,
although they usually leave behind a few
small offsets which will flower in another
four years or so. A spectacular plant for a
shady site.

Crinum x *powellii* (crinum)
2 1/2 ft (75 cm) high. Produces fragrant, rose-
pink, trumpet-like flowers in late summer.
The leaves are rather ugly and so the bulbs
are best planted among other plants. Plant
with the bulb's tall neck just above the
ground level.

Crocus
Up to 6 in (15 cm) high. Some species are
scented; the best are *C. chrysanthus* for spring
and *C. speciosus* for autumn. They do well in
full sun. Good for window boxes.

Cyclamen
6 in (15 cm) high. The two hardy cyclamen that are scented are pink- or white-flowered *C. hederifolium* (late summer and autumn) and the deep pink *C. purpurascens* in summer; the former is the more commonly grown. They are among the few bulbs that will grow in dry shade.

Galanthus (snowdrop)
6 in (15 cm) high. Most snowdrops have a faint scent on a warm day but some can be quite fragrant. *G. nivalis imperati* 'Ginns' is the most powerful and will perfume a large area. *G.* 'S. Arnott' also has a strong fragrance. They prefer light shade.

Hyacinthoides non-scriptus (English bluebell)
12 in (30 cm) high. Beautiful blue flowers, especially when grown in drifts. The Spanish bluebell is paler and has little scent compared to the English. Flowers in spring and grows best in shade. Good for planting under deciduous shrubs.

Hyacinthus (hyacinth)
12 in (30 cm) high. Club-shaped spikes of horizontally-held bluebell-like flowers in a wide variety of colors. The older varieties are the better scented. Grow in the sun. Good for window boxes or containers.

Lilium (lily)
Up to 6 ft (1.8 m) high. Many lilies and their hybrids are scented. They flower throughout the summer and come in a wide range of flower shapes and colors, from pure white to red. Not all have attractive scents; *L. pyrenaicum*, for example, smells of foxes. Most grow in full sun or light shade and thrive among other plants or in containers.

Muscari (grape hyacinth)
8 in (20 cm) high. Spikes of densely packed blue flowers that soon form a thick carpet. Flowers appear in spring and are honey-scented. The leaves are a bit unsightly. Plant in sun.

Narcissus (daffodil)
Up to 20 in (50 cm) high. Most are scented but some more sweetly so than others, especially the smaller-flowered species. *N. poeticus recurvus*, the old pheasant's eye narcissus, is one of the most delightfully fragrant. They grow in sun or light shade and flower in the late winter and spring. Good for window boxes and containers.

Tulipa (tulips)
Up to 2 ½ ft (75 cm) high. Many have a distinctive scent but usually only at close proximity. They come in a wide variety of colors and flower in the spring. Useful for bedding schemes, containers. and growing among perennials. Grow in sun.

TREES AND SHRUBS

Many trees and shrubs have fragrant flowers, often produced in such quantities as to perfume the air for some distance around. A few have fragrant leaves, but these are mainly herbs, such as thyme, sage, and rosemary (see above). Climbing shrubs are also considered separately (see below).

Because trees and shrubs will be in the ground for some time, it pays to prepare the soil thoroughly. Dig in plenty of well-rotted organic material and remove all perennial weeds. Few trees and shrubs like to grow in waterlogged conditions, so ensure that the area to be planted is well-drained.

Plant in autumn or spring at any time that the weather and soil are suitable. Plant to the same depth as the tree or shrub was in its container or nursery bed. Support, especially in windy areas, by inserting a stake beside the plant (preferably before it is planted to avoid piercing the roots). Fasten the stem to the stake with a rubber tree tie that will not chafe the bark. The tie should be about 12 in (30 cm) above ground.

Few trees, but some shrubs, need pruning. As a general rule, prune shrubs after flowering; remove about a third of the new growth. Some plants (lilac, for example) look better if the old flower heads are removed once they have finished flowering. Top-dress around trees and shrubs with organic material every autumn and spring.

Azara dentata (azara)
Up to 12 ft (3.5 m) high. Evergreen. A tender shrub that likes to be sited against a warm wall. It produces tufts of deliciously-scented, golden-yellow flowers in the spring. Plant in full sun, but it will take light shade.

Berberis (barberry)
Up to 10 ft (3 m) high. Evergreen/ deciduous. A large group of plants; a few are honey-scented. Flowers range from pale yellow to orange. *B. x stenophylla*, which is covered in fragrant yellow flowers in spring, is one of the best. Many have spines.

Buddleia (buddleia, butterfly bush)
Up to 15 ft (4.5 m) high. Deciduous. A popular genus of fragrant shrubs that are often grown for their attraction to butterflies. Flower color varieties from lilac to purple and includes white and yellow. Flowers from summer into autumn. Most need cutting almost to the ground each spring. Prefer a warm, sunny position.

Chimonanthus praecox (wintersweet)
Up to 8 ft (2.5 m) high. Deciduous. A winter-flowering shrub with a very strong scent coming from the yellowish flowers that cover the bare stems. Does best in full sun but will tolerate a little shade.

Choisya ternata (Mexican orange blossom)
Up to 6 ft (1.8 m) high. Evergreen. A rounded bush with glossy green foliage and clusters of white, star-like flowers that produce a wonderful orange-blossom scent in late spring and into summer. Prefers a sunny position, but will flower in light shade.

Cistus (rock rose)
Up to 4 ft (1.2 m) high. Evergreen. The leaves and buds of these shrubs have a powerful resinous scent. Each flower only lasts for a day, but there is a long succession of flowers through early and mid-summer. Likes full sun and a well-drained position.

Clerodendrum (glory-bower)
Up to 12 ft (3.5 m) high. Deciduous. Ambivalent plants with sweet-smelling flowers in late summer, but the foliage is unattractively fetid if bruised. Flowers are pink in the shorter *C. bungei* and white in the taller, more tree-like *C. trichotomum*. The former does best in sun while the latter prefers light shade.

Corylopsis
Up to 12 ft (3.5 m) high. Deciduous. Late winter-flowering shrub with pale yellow, hanging flowers on the bare branches. Prefers a lightly shaded position.

Daphne
Up to 5 ft (1.5 m) high. Evergreen/semi-evergreen. These shrubs vary from ground-hugging forms for the rock garden to bigger varieties for the rest of the garden. All have a delicious, heady scent. Most have pink flowers, which are produced from late winter into early summer, depending on the species. Prefer light shade or sun.

Drimys winteri
Up to 13 ft (4 m) high. Evergreen. Small trees or large shrubs that are slightly tender, so do best with wall protection. Leathery leaves and bunches of white, fragrant flowers in spring. The shrubby *D. lanceolata* has aromatic foliage.

Elaeagnus
Up to 12 ft (3.5 m) high. Evergreen/deciduous. A genus of shrubs usually grown for foliage, but also blessed with beautifully scented flowers. Flowering time varies from early summer to autumn depending on the species. Many will grow in sun or light shade.

Erica arborea (heath)
Up to 6 ft (1.8 m) high. Evergreen. A tall heather covered with masses of honey-scented flowers in spring. Heaths must have an acid soil and be grown in sun.

Eucryphia
Up to 33 ft (10 m) high. Evergreen. Trees and large shrubs that carry white cup-shaped flowers with a central boss of stamens and a honey-like scent. They flower in summer. Must be planted out of the wind, because the leaves scorch badly. Light shade is ideal.

Genista aetnensis (Mount Etna broom)
Up to 15 ft (4.5 m) high. Deciduous. Shrub or small tree with tumbling branches covered in a cascade of yellow flowers that waft sweet scent for some distance around. Needs a sunny position and not too rich a soil.

Hamamelis (witch hazel)
Up to 15 ft (4.5 m) high. Deciduous. A large group of plants with bunches of strap-like flowers that appear in late winter before the branches are clothed in leaves. They are mainly yellow but there are darker forms that tend toward orange and red. Will grow in sun but prefer a light shade.

Itea ilicifolia
Up to 10 ft (3 m) tall. Evergreen. A wall shrub with glossy leaves and long tassels of white, honey-scented flowers that appear in late summer. Prefers a sunny or lightly shaded position.

Magnolia
Up to 30 ft (9 m) high. Deciduous. Trees and shrubs, some of which have scented flowers in the spring to late summer depending on species. Most grow in sun or light shade.

Mahonia (Oregon grape)
Up to 10 ft (3 m) high. Evergreen. Winter-flowering shrubs with spiny, leather-textured foliage and spikes of very fragrant yellow flowers. Look best mixed with other plants and are useful for shady areas, although they will grow in sun.

Myrtus communis (myrtle)
Up to 10 ft (3 m) high. Evergreen. Slightly tender shrub that does best with wall protection. In autumn it is covered with white flowers that are distinctly fragrant. Grow in a warm sunny spot.

Osmanthus
Up to 10 ft (3 m) high. Evergreen. Popular shrubs with clusters of highly fragrant white flowers that perfume the air for a long way around. All are spring-flowering except *O. heterophyllus* and *O. armatus*, which flower in autumn. Grow in sun or light shade.

Philadelphus (mock orange)
Up to 12 ft (3.5 m) high. Deciduous. A large group of shrubs with white flowers that have a distinctive fragrance in late spring to early summer. Grow in sun or light shade.

Rhododendron luteum
Up to 8 ft (2.5 m) high. Deciduous. Several rhododendrons have scented flowers but this azalea is one of the best. It has yellow flowers that perfume the air for a long way around. Does best in light shade but will grow in sun.

Ribes odoratum (clove currant)
Up to 7 ft (2 m) high. Deciduous. A bright green leaved shrub with golden yellow flowers perfuming the air with cloves. The flowering currant (*R. sanguineum*) has a distinct foxy smell that comes from its leaves. Both will grow in sun or light shade.

Rosa (rose)
Up to 10 ft (3 m) high. Deciduous/semi-evergreen. Not all roses are scented, but a great number are, especially the old-fashioned shrub roses. Older varieties, however, tend to only flower once in a season. A few have scented leaves, especially noticeable after rain. Plant in full sun.

Santolina (lavender cotton)
Up to 18 in (45 cm) high. Evergreen. Attractive, feathery, gray foliage has a distinct aromatic scent when bruised or brushed against. Plant in full sun.

Syringa (lilac)
Up to 15 ft (4.5 m) high. Deciduous. These shrubs or small trees are one of the glories of spring with their lilac flowers (also white, purple, and pink) that produce a distinctive scent. Plant in a sunny position.

CLIMBERS

Some of the scented climbers below are self-supporting, but others can scramble up through trees and bushes and need to be tied in if trained over poles or wires. The ground should be well prepared before planting, which should be during the winter months. Tie in to a cane leading to the supports and continue to tie in stray stems.

Clematis
Up to 25 ft (7.5 m) high. Clings with tendrils. Most of the large-flowered hybrids are not scented, but a number of the smaller-flowered species are fragrant. Most of these do not require pruning except to contain them if they get too large. Plant with the roots in shade and top in sunshine.

Humulus lupulus (common hop)
15 ft (4.5 m) high. Climbs by twining. The female flowers (hops) have a distinctive aromatic scent. Plant in sun or light shade.

Jasminum (jasmine)
15 ft (4.5 m) high. Scrambles, needs tying in. White, pink, or yellow flowers with a sweet evening scent. Plant in sun.

Lonicera (honeysuckle)
Up to 20 ft (6 m) high. Climbs by twining. Not all are scented. From spring to summer they produce whorls of yellow and pink flowers that are highly scented, especially in the evening. Plant in shade or sun.

Rosa (climbing roses, rambling roses)
Up to 30 ft (9 m) high. Climb by scrambling and will need to be tied in. A wide range of colors from white and yellow to pink and red. Some flower more than once in a season. Not all are scented. Plant in sun.

Wisteria
Up to 25 ft (7.5 m) high. Climbs by scrambling and twining and will need to be tied in. Long tassels of lilac or white flowers with a pervasive, delicate fragrance. Prune rigorously for good flowering.

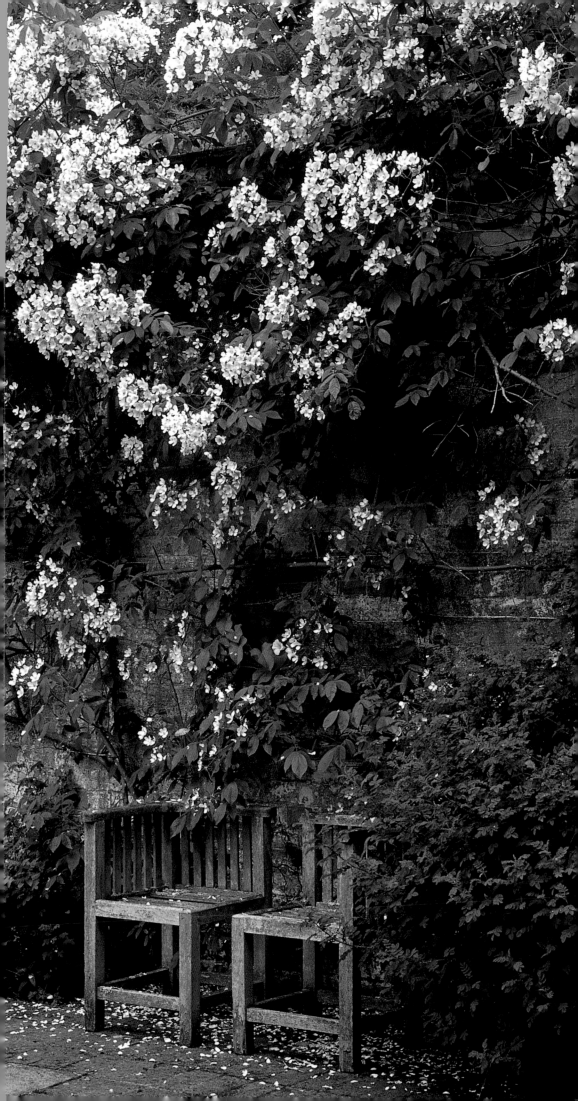

useful addresses

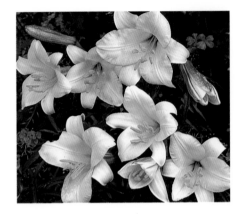

Plants, seeds and trees

Adams County Nursery, Inc.
P.O. Box 10826
Nursery Lane
Aspers, PA 17304
www.acnursery.com

Dacha Barinka
46232 Strathcona Road
Chilliwack, BC,
Canada V2P 3T2
(604) 792-0957

W. Atlee Burpee & Company
300 Park Avenue
Warminster, PA 18974-0001
(800) 888-1447
www.burpee.com

Carroll Gardens
444 E. Main Street
Westminster, MD 21157
(800) 638-6334

Companion Plants
7247 N. Coolville Ridge Road,
Athens, OH 45701
(740) 592-4643
www.frognet.net/companion–
plants

Dabney Herbs
P.O. Box 22061
Louisville, KY 40252
(502) 893-5198
www.dabneyherbs.com

**Eden Organic Nursery
Services, Inc.**
P.O. Box 4604
Hallandale, FL 33008
(954) 455-0229
www.eonseed.com

Four Winds Growers
P.O. Box 3538
Fremont, CA 94539
www.fourwindsgrowers.com

The Fragrant Path
P.O. Box 328
Ft. Calhoun, NE 68023-0328

Good Scents
1308 N. Meridian Road
Meridian, ID 83642
(208) 887-1784
http://netnow.micron.net/~basil

Garden City Seeds
778 Highway 93 North
Hamilton, MT 59840
(406) 961-4837

It's About Thyme
11726 Manchaca Road
Austin, TX 78748
(512) 280-1192
http://mvpimages.net/itsthyme

Island Seed Company
P.O. Box 4278, Depot 3
Victoria, BC,
Canada V8X 3X8

Johnny's Selected Seeds
Route 1, Box 2580, Foss Hill Road
Albion, ME 04910-9731
(207) 437-9294
www.johnnyseeds.com

Henry Leuthardt Nurseries, Inc.,
P.O. Box 666
Montauk Highway
East Moriches, NY 11940
(516) 878-1387

Mellinger's
2310 W. South Range Road
North Lima, OH 44452

**Santa Barbara Heirloom
Nursery, Inc.**
P.O. Box 4235
Santa Barbara, CA 93140-4235
(805) 968-5444
www.heirloom.com

Seeds of Change
P.O. Box 15700
Santa Fe, NM 87506-5700
(888) 762-7333
www.seedsofchange.com

Shepherd's Garden Seeds
30 Irene Street
Torrington, CT 06790
(860) 496-9624, 482-3638
www.shepherdseeds.com

Southern Exposure Seed
Exchange, P.O. Box170
Earlysville, VA 22936
(804) 973-4703
www.southernexposure.com

Story House Herb Farm
587 Erwin Road
Murray, KY 42071
(502) 753-4158

Wayside Gardens
1 Garden Lane
Hodges, SC 29695-0001
(800) 845-1124

West Coast Seeds, Inc.
8475 Ontario Street, Unit 206
Vancouver, BC,
Canada V5X 3E8
(604) 482-8800
www.westcoastseeds.com

Arbors, ornaments, and trellises

Bow Bends
P.O. Box 900
Bolton, MA 01740-0900
(508) 779-6464

Cincinnati Artistic Wrought Iron
2943 Eastern Avenue
Cincinnati, OH 45226

Garden Arches
P.O. Box 4057-B
Bellingham, WA 98227

The Garden Architecture Group
631 North Third Street
Philadelphia, PA 19123

Garden Concepts, Inc.
P.O. Box 241233
Memphis, TN 38124-1233
(901) 756-1649

Garden Trellises, Inc.
P.O. Box 105
LaFayette, NY 13084-0105
(315) 498-9003
www.GardenTrellises.com

Heritage Garden Furnishings and Curios
1209 E. Island Highway, 6
Parksville, BC
Canada V9P 1R5
(250) 248-9598

The Home Depot
for nearest store, contact:
(800) 430-3376 (US)
(800) 668-2266 (CAN)
www.HomeDepot.com

Kinsman Company, Inc.
P.O. Box 357,
Old Firehouse, River Road
Point Pleasant, PA 18950
(800) 733-4146
www.kinsmangarden.com

Smith & Hawken
P.O. Box 6907
Florence, KY 41022-6900
(800) 777-5858
www.Smith-Hawken.com

Stillbrook Horticultural Supplies
P.O. Box 600
Bantam, CT 06750-0600
(800) 414-4468
www.stillbrook.com

Sumerset Arbors
P.O. Box 7243
Beaumont, TX 77726-7243
(800) 645-3391

credits

The publishers would like to thank the following garden owners and designers for allowing their gardens to be photographed:

Barry Road, London SE22, Jonathan & Sam Buckley; Brodrick Road, London SW17, Helen Yemm; Burbage Road, London SE24, Rosemary Lindsay; Chenies Manor, Buckinghamshire, Mrs Macleod-Matthews; Cinque Cottage, Sussex, Julian Upston; Clinton Lodge, Sussex, Mr & Mrs Collum; Eglatine Road, London, Janie Lloyd Owen; Great Dixter, East Sussex, Christopher Lloyd; Hollington Nurseries, Berkshire, Simon & Judith Hopkinson; Marle Place, Kent, Mr & Mrs Williams; Old Place Farm, Kent, Mr & Mrs Jeffrey Eker; RHS Gardens, Wisley; Roger's Rough, Kent, Richard & Hilary Bird; Rommany Road, London, Belinda Barnes & Ronald Stuart-Moonlight; Royal Botanic Gardens, Kew; Stockton Bury, Herefordshire, Gordon Fenn & Raymond Treasure; The Anchorage, West Wickham, Kent, Wendy Francis; The Herb Farm, Reading, Berkshire; Upper Mill Cottage, Kent, David & Mavis Seeney; West Dean Gardens, Sussex, Edward James Foundation.

Jonathan Buckley would particularly like to thank Judith and Simon Hopkinson at Hollington Nurseries for their help throughout this project.

index

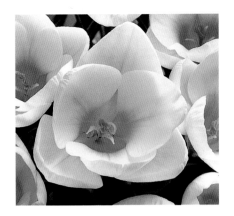

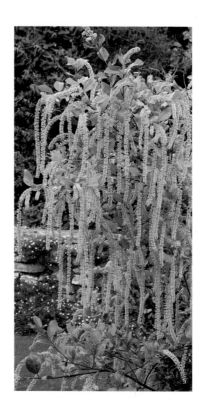

acknowledgments

The author would like to thank all those involved in bringing this book to fruition: Anne Ryland whose idea it was and who commissioned me to write it; Marek Walisiewicz for his editing and suggestions; Paul Reid for his design, which brings the whole thing to life; the illustrator, Sally Launder, who has gone to great pains to turn rough sketches into images; and last, but not least, Jonathan Buckley whose brilliant photographs make the book.

Thanks also go to all the owners who allowed Jonathan to photograph their wonderful scented gardens for this book.